UNDER THE FIG LEAF

ANGELO S. PAOLA, M.D.

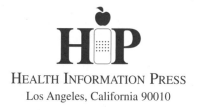

HEALTH INFORMATION PRESS

Los Angeles, California 90010

Library of Congress Cataloging-in-Publication Data

Paola, Angelo S.
    Under the fig leaf: a comprehensive guide to the care & maintenance of the
penis, prostate and related organs / Angelo S. Paola.
        p.   cm.
    Includes bibliographical references and index.
    ISBN 1-885987-15-3
    1. Generative organs, Male--Diseases--Popular works. 2. Men--Health and
hygiene--Popular works. I. Title.
RC881.P22   1998   98-39340
616.6'5--DC21   CIP

Disclaimer:
The information presented in this book is based on the experience and interpretation
of the author. Although the information has been carefully researched and checked
for accuracy, currency and completeness, neither the author nor the publisher accept
any responsibility or liability with regard to errors, omissions, misuse or misinter-
pretation.

ISBN: 1-885987-15-3

Printed in the United States of America

Health Information Press
4727 Wilshire Blvd., Suite 300
Los Angeles, CA 90010
1-800-MED-SHOP
email: MEDICALBOOKSTORE.COM

For Nick, Joe, Elle and Tony

ACKNOWLEDGEMENTS

To my parents, who instilled in me the desire to learn and to always try to do better . . .

To my teachers and professors, especially those at West Virginia University, who gave me the foundation of knowledge upon which to build. . .

To Wanda Carmenate and Manuel Sierra who helped me overcome my computer ignorance in the preparation of this manuscript. . .

To Kathryn Swanson, Maureen Lynch and Health Information Press who helped get this work published. . .

And last, but not least, to my wife, Brigitte, without whose support and apparently infinite understanding this book would never have been completed. . .

I wish to express my deepest gratitude. . . I could never have done this without all of you.

Angelo S. Paola, M.D.

TABLE OF CONTENTS

PREFACE

After a few years in practice, I became aware that there were questions regarding certain urologic problems that were extremely common among my patients. I also began to note that there weren't many places that a person could go to find the answers, other than a urologist's office. Not to be chauvinistic, but although bookstores have areas devoted to women's health issues, I could rarely find any information for the general public regarding men's health issues. True, there are some magazines which deal with men's health, but over time, I began to feel that there may be need for a book that focuses on the common urologic problems that can affect a man as he goes through life and attempts to address some of the common questions and misconceptions regarding these problems. And so, I decided to write *Under the Fig Leaf: A Comprehensive Guide to the Care & Maintenance of the Penis, Prostate and Related Organs.*

I have attempted to arrange the topics in the order that they are roughly seen in a man's life —from birth to old age, or as close as possible to that time sequence, except for the chapters dealing with urologic cancers. I also tried to present the material without a lot of medical mumbo-jumbo. However, in a book of this type, a certain amount of medical terminology is unavoidable. I have attempted to clarify these terms whenever possible.

In each chapter, I tried to discuss the topic with regard to cause, diagnosis, and treatment options, and I also attempted to answer some of the more common questions that I'm asked about each problem by the patients I see in my office. As a result, I hope that after reading this book, men and their partners will have a better understanding of certain urologic health issues.

The actor Wilson Mizner once said, "when you steal from one author, it is called plagiarism; if you steal from many, it is research." Most of the information in this book is not the result of my own original thought processes. It was gathered over years of study and training, and was originally obtained by researchers much more knowledgeable than myself.

It should be noted that this book is not meant to replace a urologic evaluation! After all, I don't want to put myself out of business... However, I feel there may be people who are too embarrassed to ask questions about certain urologic problems. Hopefully, this book may help to answer some of those questions, or at least, show people that they are not alone. And maybe, as a result, it may prompt them to seek medical attention for a problem sooner, rather than ignoring a symptom that could come back to haunt them later on.

GLOSSARY

Abscess: A localized collection of pus.

Acquired: That which develops during life, as opposed to congenital.

Adjuvant therapy: A type of treatment used in addition to the main form of treatment.

AID: Artificial insemination of a female with donor semen.

AIH: Artificial insemination of a female with her husband's semen.

Alpha blockers: Drugs that relax the muscles in and around the prostate in order to help relieve the symptoms of benign prostatic hyperplasia (BPH).

Amyloidosis: A condition in which a wax-like protein builds up in various organs of the body, routinely the liver and kidneys.

Analgesic: A medicine which relieves pain.

Anastomosis: The site where two structures are connected after an organ has been removed.

Androgens: Hormones secreted predominantly by the testicles or synthetic substances which control the build-up of protein and the male secondary sex characteristics (e.g., distribution of hair and deepening of the voice). Hence the name, *male hormones*.

Anemia: Abnormally low red blood cell count which could be a sign of internal bleeding or cancer.

Antibiotics: A drug used to fight infection.

Anticoagulant: A substance that prevents the blood from clotting, frequently called a blood thinner. Examples include heparin, aspirin, Coumadin, and ibuprofen.

Arteriography: A dye test used to study blood flow in arteries, especially used in the evaluation of some patients with impotence.

Asymptomatic: Symptomless, or having no symptoms.

Atherosclerosis: Degenerative change in the arteries that is associated with aging.

Atrophic: Smaller in size and function than usual (as in an *atrophic* testicle).

Autologous blood donation: A procedure in which patients donate their own blood before surgery for the specific purpose of having it available in case they need a transfusion during or after surgery.

Azoospermia: Lack of any sperm in the semen.

Benign: A term that means non-cancerous.

Benign prostatic hyperplasia (BPH): Non-cancerous enlargement of the prostate that often occurs in older men. While benign, it can cause obstruction of the urethra and difficulty in urinating.

Bladder: A muscular structure situated in the pelvis that holds urine until a person is ready to urinate.

Bladder neck: The part of the bladder that opens into the urethra (i.e., where the bladder meets the urethra).

Blood thinner: See *Anticoagulant.*

Body habitus: Referring to a patient's build or size.

BPH: see *Benign prostatic hyperplasia.*

Cancer: A general term used to describe many malignant growths in many parts of the body. In this disease, cell growth is out of control.

Catheter: A hollow tube that is inserted up the urethra to drain urine from the bladder. If the catheter is to stay in the bladder for any period of time, a balloon at the end of the catheter is inflated to prevent the catheter from falling out.

Cavernosonography: An x-ray test in which contrast dye is injected into the penis to visualize the corpora cavernosa and to search for venous leaks.

Chemotherapy: The use of drugs to kill cancer cells.

Coagulopathy: A problem with the blood that prevents its normal ability to form clots or solidify, which manifests itself as a tendency to bleed easily and for prolonged periods of time.

Color flow Doppler: A diagnostic test that uses ultrasound to detect and visualize blood flow in an organ. This test can be very useful in evaluating for the presence of testicular torsion.

Congenital: Present at birth.

Contralateral: Situated on, or pertaining to, the opposite side.

Corpora cavernosa: The paired cylindrical chambers of the penis which fill with blood during erection.

Corporus spongiusum: The spongy tissue on the underside of the penis through which runs the urethra.

Creatinine: A chemical in the blood which can be measured by a blood test and is used to evaluate a person's kidney function.

Cryotherapy: A procedure that uses very cold temperatures to destroy cancerous tissues.

Cyst: A fluid-filled sac which is usually benign. For example, renal cysts are present in 50 percent of patients over the age of fifty. They are usually of no clinical significance.

Cystoscope: An instrument which uses fiberoptic light to see into the urethra and bladder.

Cystoscopy: A procedure which involves the use of a fiberoptic instrument to view the urethra, prostate, and bladder.

Detorsion: In the case of testicular torsion, untwisting of the spermatic cord to reestablish blood flow to the testicle.

Diabetes mellitus: A medical problem characterized by elevation of blood sugar levels due to a deficiency or diminished effectiveness of insulin.

Diuretics: Drugs that increase urine production (commonly known as "water pills").

DNA (deoxyribonucleic acid): Structure that is part of every cell. It carries the blueprints or code for living tissue; i.e., the building block of life. Problems with DNA can lead to birth defects or predispose a person to cancer.

Dysuria: Burning or uncomfortable sensation on urination.

Embryo: Term applied to the developing human in the first eight weeks of pregnancy.

Endocrine: Pertaining to hormones.

Enuresis: Urinary incontinence in children. Typically known as *bed wetting*.

Epididymis: The convoluted structure attached to the testicle where sperm are stored and mature. It eventually straightens out to become the vas deferens.

Erectile dysfunction: Inability to achieve or maintain erections adequate enough for vaginal penetration and sexual satisfaction (also called *impotence*).

Estrogens: Female hormones. These are present in small quantities in males.

Fascia: A sheath of fibrous tissue and fat which unites the skin to the underlying tissue. It also surrounds and separates muscles and some organs.

FDA: See *Food and Drug Administration.*

Fistula: An abnormal communication between two cavities or body surfaces.

Flank: The area of the back and side that is lateral to the spine and at the level of the lower ribs.

Foley catheter: See *Catheter.*

Follicle stimulating hormone: A hormone which stimulates sperm production in the testicles.

Food and Drug Administration: Also called the FDA, this federal agency approves drugs and treatments for public use.

Frequency: Term used to describe abnormally frequent urination. In this case, the patient urinates frequently (i.e., every one to two hours), but not much urine is elicited each time.

FSH: See *Follicle stimulating hormone.*

Genitalia: The organs responsible for reproduction (the sex organs). In the male, these include the penis and testicles.

Germ cells: Cells in the testicle that give rise to sperm.

Glans penis: The bulbous end of the penis, also known as the head of the penis.

Gynecomastia: Enlargement of breast tissue which can be seen in men with certain types of testicular cancer or in men who undergo certain types of hormone therapy for prostate cancer.

Hematocele: Collection of blood around the testicle, usually the result of trauma.

Hematoma: A localized collection of blood.

Hesitancy: Difficulty starting urine flow.

High blood pressure (HBP): See *Hypertension.*

Hormone: A chemical that controls various bodily functions.

Hypercalciuria: Elevated levels of calcium in the urine. This has been associated with kidney stone formation.

Hypertension: Blood pressure elevation beyond the accepted normal values. This condition may increase the risk of heart attack and stroke.

Hyperuricosuria: Elevated levels of uric acid in the urine. This condition may also increase the risk of kidney stone formation.

Iatrogenic: Resulting from a physician or medicine.

Idiopathic: A condition of unknown origin (no known cause).

Immunotherapy: Any treatment used to stimulate the immune system to fight disease.

Impotence: See *Erectile dysfunction.*

Incision: A cut made by a surgeon to get to the structure that needs to be removed or repaired.

Inguinal: Pertaining to the area of the lower part of the abdomen just above the beginning of the thigh on each side (also known as the groin area).

Incidence: The number of new cases of a specific disease occurring during a certain period of time.

Incubation period: The time from entry of infection to the appearance of the first symptom.

Interferons: Naturally occurring proteins used to stimulate the immune system to fight disease.

Intravenous: Placed into a vein.

Intravenous pyelogram (IVP): An x-ray study in which dye injected intravenously is filtered by the kidneys and used to visualize the kidneys, ureter, and bladder.

In vitro fertilization (IVF): Technique used to achieve a pregnancy in which sperm and the female egg are manipulated outside the body (as in a test tube).

Ipsilateral: Situated on, or pertaining to, the same side.

Ischemia: Lack of blood supply to an organ.

Kidneys: Two organs situated on each side of the spine in the upper posterior abdominal cavity whose job it is to filter toxins from the blood which are then excreted into the urine.

KUB: An x-ray looking at the area of the kidneys, ureters, and bladder, especially to evaluate for the presence of stones.

Latency time: Duration of intravaginal contact or the number of thrusts before ejaculation.

Latent period: See *Refractory period.*

LH: See *Luteinizing hormone.*

LHRH: See *Luteinizing hormone releasing hormone.*

LHRH agonist: A synthetic hormone that is similar to LHRH which is used to treat prostate cancer. When given as a drug, LHRH agonists inhibit the production of testosterone by the testicles.

Libido: The sexual urge or sex drive.

Ligate: To tie off.

Luteinizing hormone: A chemical produced by the pituitary gland that stimulates testosterone production in the testicles.

Luteinizing hormone releasing hormone: A chemical produced by the brain that stimulates the release of luteinizing hormone by the pituitary gland.

Lymph nodes: Oval structures made up of lymphocytes (infection fighting cells) that are located throughout the body. When cancer escapes from an organ, one of the first places it spreads to is nearby lymph nodes.

Malignant: A term that means cancerous.

Meatus: An opening, as in urethral meatus.

Metastasis: The spread of cancer beyond its organ of origin to other sites in the body.

Micturition: The act of urination.

Nocturia: Waking up at night to urinate. This could be a symptom of prostate problems.

Nocturnal penile tumescence (NPT): Erections during sleep. Studies of this phenomenon in the laboratory setting are called NPT studies and may be used in the work up of erectile dysfunction.

Nuclear medicine testicular scan: A diagnostic test in which radioactive chemicals are injected intravenously and followed by a machine that detects radioactivity to evaluate for the presence of blood flow to the testicles. This test is used in the evaluation for possible torsion.

Oligospermia: Fewer than the normal number of sperm on a semen analysis.

Orchiectomy: The surgical removal of a testicle. Bilateral orchiectomy, the removal of both testicles, also known as castration, is one treatment option for advanced or metastatic prostate cancer.

Orchiopexy: Placing and fixing the testicle in the scrotum.

Paraphimosis: Condition in which the retracted foreskin of the penis is trapped behind the glans, resulting in pain, swelling and inflammation.

Pathognomonic: Characteristic of, or peculiar to, a disease.

Pathologist: A doctor who examines the tissues and cells of the body under a microscope to determine what type of disease is present.

Pediatric urologist: A urologist trained to specialize in urologic problems occurring in children.

Pelvic area: The area of the body below the waist containing the bladder, prostate, rectum, and sexual organs.

Penile: Pertaining to the penis.

Penile duplex Doppler ultrasound: A diagnostic study that uses sound waves to study penile blood flow.

Percutaneous: Through unbroken skin. For example, many urologic procedures are done *percutaneously* by making a small hole in the skin and then using laparoscopic instruments to work inside the body rather than by cutting the patient open to operate on a particular organ.

Perineum: The area between the scrotum and the anus.

Periurethral glands: Small glands that surround the urethra. They produce fluids to help lubricate the urethra during the sexual act.

Phantom pain: Discomfort perceived as coming from an organ that has been removed. For example, some patients feel pain in a leg even after it has been cut off to treat disease.

Pharmacologic: Pertaining to drugs.

Pharmacotherapy: The use of drugs to treat medical problems.

Phimosis: Narrowing or constriction of the distal penile foreskin which prevents its normal retraction over the glans penis.

Phytotherapy: The use of plants and plant extracts for medicinal purposes.

Pituitary gland: A small organ located in the brain that is involved in the regulation of hormones throughout the body.

Placebo: A harmless substance given as a medicine, like a sugar pill. In some experimental studies one group of patients will get the real medicine and the other will get the placebo. The placebo is used to evaluate the effectiveness of the real medication.

Prognosis: An estimation of the probable course and termination of a disease.

Prostate: An accessory sex gland located just below the bladder and through which passes the urethra.

Prostatic urethra: The part of the urethra that passes through the prostate.

Prostatism: The term used to describe the group of symptoms that may result from benign prostatic hyperplasia (BPH).

Radiographic: Involving the use of x-rays to image parts of the body.

Radiolucent: Not well seen on x-ray (as in certain kidney stones).

Radio-opaque: Well seen on x-ray (as in certain kidney stones).

Rectum: The lower part of the large intestines that ends at the anus.

Recurrence: When something (for example, a cancer) returns after initial treatment.

Refractory period: Also called latent period, that time after ejaculation during which another erection is not possible. The duration of this increases with increasing age.

REM sleep (rapid eye movement sleep): That part of the sleep cycle during which people dream and which is associated with nocturnal erections.

Renal: Pertaining to the kidney.

RPR (rapid plasma reagin): A blood test for syphilis.

Retroperitoneum: That part of the body located behind the abdominal cavity and containing the kidneys, adrenal glands, and the major blood vessels (i.e., the aorta and the inferior vena cava).

Risk factor: Something that increases a person's chances of getting a disease.

Scrotum: The pouch of skin below the penis that holds the testicles and spermatic cord.

Secondary sex characteristics: Changes in appearance due to "sex hormones." For example, in males these are changes seen in response to androgens (such as distribution of hair and deepening of the voice).

Semen analysis: Examination of the seminal fluid.

Seminal vesicles: Accessory sex glands situated near the prostate which store sperm and also produce nutrients for the sperm to use after ejaculation.

Spermatic cord: The structure that suspends the testicle in the scrotum and which contains the blood supply of the testicle as well as the vas deferens.

Spermatogenesis: The production of sperm.

Spermicide: A chemical that is toxic to sperm.

Steinstrasse: From German meaning "street of stones." A condition in which fragments from kidney stones treated with ESWL pass into the ureter causing obstruction and pain.

Stricture: A narrowing due to scar tissue.

Sulfasalazine: A drug used to treat inflammatory bowel diseases, such as ulcerative colitis and Crohn's disease.

Symptomatic: Term used to describe a patient who is feeling the effects of a disease.

Testicles (testes): The paired organs in the scrotum which produce sperm and most of the body's testosterone.

Testosterone: The male hormone produced predominantly by the testicles, which is responsible for male secondary sex characteristics. Some testosterone is produced by the adrenal glands.

Torsion: Twisting (as in twisting of the spermatic cord which can result in damage to the testicles).

Transillumination: The transmission of light for diagnostic purposes.

Tumor: An abnormal growth that can be benign or malignant.

Ultrasound: A diagnostic test that produces a visual image by using sound waves inaudible to the human ear for the purpose of visualizing internal organs.

Ureter: The tube that carries urine from the kidney to the bladder.

Urethra: The tube passing through the penis and through which urine and semen travel to get out of the body.

Urethral meatus: Opening in the penis where the urine comes out.

Urethral sphincter: The muscles that are responsible for urinary continence. They are located at the bladder neck and at the bottom of the prostate.

Urethral stricture: A narrowing of the urethra due to scar tissue.

Urgency: The feeling of having to urinate immediately.

Urinalysis (U/A): Examination of the urine.

Urinary retention: The inability to urinate. It may be due to obstruction (for example, by an enlarged prostate, prostate cancer, or urethral stricture) or due to a weak bladder muscle.

Urologist: A surgeon who specializes in problems with the kidneys, bladder, prostate, and the male sexual organs.

Varicocelectomy: Surgical repair of a varicocele.

Vas deferens: The tube that carries sperm from the epididymis to the urethra (pleural form is *vasa deferentia*).

VDRL: A blood test for syphilis.

Voiding cystourethrogram (VCUG): An x-ray study in which, after contrast dye is injected into the bladder via a catheter inserted in the urethra, pictures are taken while the patient urinates to search for abnormalities (e.g., strictures or sources of infection).

Watchful waiting: A treatment option in which a person diagnosed with prostate cancer decides to carefully monitor the progress of his disease with frequent follow-up rather than have immediate treatment of his disease.

CHAPTER 1

CIRCUMCISION

Circumcision, the removal of the foreskin of the penis, has been practiced for as long as man could say, "Ouch!" Its first recorded description dates back to 3000 B.C. Egypt, and it is still the most common operation performed in the United States.

There are three basic indications for circumcision: tradition, cosmetic preference, and therapeutic need. In many cultures and societies, circumcision is viewed as a rite of passage —either religious or social. The age at which circumcision is performed varies between cultures, and can even vary within the same culture.

In cultures where circumcision is practiced commonly, women may find the uncircumcised penis ugly. While it's true that beauty is subjective, the decision to not circumcise a male child in these societies may result in ridicule and/or psychological trauma.

THERAPEUTIC ADVANTAGES

Although the most common arguments in favor of neonatal circumcision have been those of custom and tradition, there have been attempts to define the objective therapeutic benefits of circumcision. In several studies, the rate of urinary tract infections in uncircumcised infants is approximately ten times greater than in circumcised males (1 to 4 percent vs. 0.1 to 0.4 percent). These studies suggest that the presence of a foreskin predisposes male infants to urinary tract infection, possibly by allowing bacteria to colonize the area around the urethral meatus, the opening in the head of the penis where the urine comes out.

Phimosis is a narrowing or constriction of the distal penile foreskin which prevents its normal retraction over the glans (i.e., head of the penis). It is most commonly acquired as a result of poor hygiene and chronic infection. It occurs in approximately 1 percent of patients over 16 years of

1

age. This needs to be differentiated from the inability to retract the foreskin during infancy which is a normal occurrence. These congenital adhesions naturally separate during the first one to three years of life. Phimosis is an indication for circumcision. Circumcision in infancy can be protective against the development of phimosis.

Paraphimosis is a condition in which the retracted foreskin remains trapped behind the glans, resulting in swelling, pain, and inflammation. Paraphimosis can also be prevented and/or treated with circumcision.

Retention of urine and smegma under the foreskin can lead to recurrent infection. Studies suggest that the dry skin of the circumcised penis is more resistant to infection. The risk of certain infections has been suggested to be lower in the circumcised penis, e.g. gonorrhea, syphilis, chancroid, warts, viral hepatitis, genital herpes, and HIV. None of the studies, however, have proven that it is better to remove the foreskin rather than just keep it clean.

On rare occasions, the foreskin may get caught in a zipper or may get torn during retraction. Circumcision may be therapeutically indicated in these instances.

Circumcision in infancy is protective against cancer of the penis. Although cancer of the penis is rare, it is almost unheard of in the circumcised penis. Only approximately 30 cases of penile cancer have been reported in males circumcised before age five.

RISKS

Circumcision is surgery and, therefore, not without risk. The complication rate of circumcision is approximately 0.2 to 5 percent. Risks of the procedure include infection, bleeding, pain, and adhesions to the head of the penis. Neonatal circumcision also predisposes to stenosis, or narrowing, of the meatus; however, apparent meatal stenosis seldom causes a problem. Reported complications have also included necrosis of the head of the penis, laceration of the scrotum, removal of the entire penile skin, urethral fistula, inclusion cysts at the circumcision line, loss of penis, and even lung abscess from aspiration of vomit due to crying during the procedure. The mortality rate from circumcision has been estimated to be approximately 1 in 500,000 cases.

TECHNIQUES

Circumcision can be performed using a variety of techniques. It has been suggested that infants may feel pain from circumcision, and in an attempt to lessen that pain, recently, the use of local anesthesia for the procedure in newborns has been encouraged.

- The Gomco is a device over which the foreskin is stretched before the excess is cut off. This device also compresses the tissues to prevent bleeding and achieve hemostasis after removal of the foreskin.

- The Plastibell is a plastic device that fits under the foreskin but over the head of the penis. The foreskin is trimmed and then tied over the plastibell. The string cuts through the foreskin over time, and the plastibell and excess foreskin usually fall off after five to seven days. Cases have been reported where the plastibell migrated onto the shaft of the penis (instead of falling off). In these situations, the device must be cut away from the penis.

- The sleeve technique uses two circumferential incisions in the foreskin approximately 1 centimeter apart and 0.5 to 1 centimeter proximal to the head of the penis. This strip of foreskin is then removed before suturing the cut ends together.

- In cases in which the foreskin cannot be retracted, a slit can be made in the midline on the top of the penis to the level of the groove behind the head of the penis. A second slit is made on the bottom of the foreskin, and then the two "wings" of excess foreskin are excised circumferentially.

- In some cases, and/or in ritualistic circumcisions, the guillotine technique can be performed. The foreskin is tracked distally. The glans (i.e., the head of the penis) is identified by palpation. Carefully avoiding the glans, the excess foreskin is removed with a scalpel or knife.

- In adult patients, instead of removing the excess foreskin, sometimes only the dorsal slit is performed to allow the patient to easily retract the foreskin for routine hygiene.

The technique employed for circumcision usually depends on the surgeon's preference and experience. If it is performed soon after birth, the procedure tends to be accomplished using devices, such as the Gomco clamp or the plastibell. In older boys, where penile vessels are of substantial size and usually cannot be sealed by such devices, the sleeve technique or other "free-hand" techniques are usually employed.

NEONATAL CIRCUMCISION

There is much controversy surrounding circumcision in neonates. The only apparent contraindications to the procedure include: 1) penile abnormality that may require the foreskin for repair; 2) an uncorrected bleeding disorder; or 3) a sick, premature infant. Aside from these contraindications, there have been no unequivocal definitive studies either in favor of or against neonatal circumcision. The American Academy of Pediatrics recently concluded that "newborn circumcision has potential medical advantages, as well as disadvantages and risks;" however, it does not officially recommend or discourage the procedure.

The final decision regarding neonatal circumcision is going to be left up to the parents. As a parent myself, I felt that neonatal circumcision was a relatively low-risk procedure that might spare my child some problems in adulthood. After three or four months of age, children are usually too big for the circumcision board and local anesthesia, and probably will require general anesthesia. In this case, I personally do not feel that the benefits of circumcision outweigh the risks of general anesthesia, and I usually suggest that the parents of these children may want to wait until their child is old enough to make his own decision regarding the procedure. I still leave the final decision to the parents.

If the decision is made not to circumcise a male infant, there must be a significant commitment to genital hygiene. Attempts to retract the foreskin before age two or three may tear natural adhesions and result in bleeding and subsequent scarring that could cause problems in the future. The parents are instructed to begin teaching their children to gently retract the foreskin for cleansing after age three.

This chapter isn't meant to answer the question of whether or not to circumcise a male infant, but, hopefully, some of the arguments presented will help parents make a more informed decision. Good luck!

4

References

1. Blandy JP, *et al.*: "Circumcision: A Continuing Controversy." *AUA Update Series* 1995; vol. 14, lesson 21.
2. Gillenwater JY, Grayhack JT, Howards SS, Duckett JW (eds.): *Adult and Pediatric Urology*, 3rd ed. St. Louis: Mosby, 1996.
3. Hinman F: *Atlas of Urologic Surgery*. Philadelphia: W.B. Saunders, 1989.
4. Walsh PC, Retik AB, Stamey TA, Vaughan ED (eds.): *Campbell's Urology*, 6th ed. Philadelphia: W.B. Saunders, 1992.

CHAPTER 2

ENURESIS

In infancy, when your bladder is full, it tries to empty itself and you urinate –on yourself or on whomever is in the way. As you get older, inhibitory nervous pathways develop so that you can store your urine until a time when it is more socially acceptable to void. From birth until about two years of age, most children are reflex voiders (i.e., when the bladder fills, they void spontaneously). Between two and four years of age, most children start to feel the need to void but usually can't hold their urine, so reflex voiding still occurs. By four years of age, most children are able to voluntarily control when they void –i.e., they are "dry."

Enuresis refers to involuntary wetting in children, and is usually taken to mean bedwetting. Primary enuresis is present from birth, and secondary enuresis is preceded by a dry interval of six to twelve months. The prevalence of enuresis in children at 5, 10, and 15 years of age is approximately 15, 5, and 1 percent respectively. Bedwetting should be viewed as a developmental delay in the inhibitory influence of the central nervous system on the urinary bladder. Other theories regarding the cause of enuresis attribute it to psychogenic and behavioral components, environmental influences, deep sleep, allergies, small bladder capacity, and true anatomic abnormalities. The finding of underlying organic problems is rare in primary enuresis, and is usually higher in the older patients. A familial predisposition for enuresis has been reported. Approximately 40 percent of children will be enuretic if one parent had the condition, and 70 percent will be enuretic if both parents were affected.

Years ago, most children who continued to wet the bed after age four or five underwent a significant evaluation with invasive studies (e.g., intravenous pyelogram (IVP), voiding cystourethrogram (VCUG), and cystoscopy). Usually, the work-up found only a lower functional bladder capacity. Since true organic pathology is rare, current recommendations call

7

for a less invasive evaluation. A thorough history and physical examination, urinalysis, urine culture, and a plain x-ray of the abdomen are generally all that are necessary for the initial evaluation. If these studies suggest a true problem, then a more thorough investigation including IVP, VCUG, and cystoscopy may be indicated.

Since spontaneous resolution can be expected in most cases of bedwetting, it is important to assess the significance of the problem on the patient and family before initiating therapy. If the initial evaluation is unremarkable, it should be understood that 1) the urinary tract is probably normal; 2) bedwetting is usually involuntary and the child should not be blamed or punished; and 3) spontaneous resolution will usually occur with toilet training and fluid restriction before bedtime as the only treatment. Spontaneous resolution usually occurs at a rate of approximately 15 percent per year in patients between 5 and 19 years of age. As the child reaches school age and social pressures increase, behavioral therapy can be considered. A conditioning device like the pad-and-bell alarm is successful in up to 60 percent of patients. When aided by positive reinforcement, behavior modification therapy which is aimed at making the child responsible for his behavior, is helpful in up to 70 percent of patients. These techniques require highly motivated children and parents; however, the positive results last longer than after drug therapy.

For patients (or their parents) who are unable to practice behavior therapy or who fail with it, drug therapy can be effective. One group of drugs attempts to relax the bladder muscle so the bladder can hold more urine at night. Some of these drugs include oxybutynin (Ditropan), and imipramine (Tofranil). Up to 70 percent of children with nocturnal enuresis are successfully treated with imipramine, with some relapses after withdrawal. Side effects of this drug include nausea, malaise, anxiety, personality changes, cardiac arrhythmias, and sleep disorders. However, these drugs are usually well tolerated.

Desmopressin acetate (DDAVP) is a drug which reduces urine production. A dose of 20 to 40 micrograms/night intranasally has been shown to be effective in decreasing or eliminating bedwetting in children and adults who have failed behavioral and other pharmacologic therapies. DDAVP seems to be more effective in children with a family history of nocturnal enuresis. Side effects include nasal stuffiness, nose bleeds, and mild abdominal pain. Recently, DDAVP has become available in oral form with a reported efficacy similar to intranasal dosing. As with other forms of drug therapy for enuresis, early withdrawal of DDAVP has been associated with a high relapse rate, particularly in younger children.

Basically, bedwetting should be viewed as a developmental delay in the inhibition to void. Unless the child has symptoms of urinary tract infection (e.g., frequent voiding, or burning with urination), voiding problems, involuntary loss of stool, abnormal urinalysis, or some other abnormality suggesting anything other than a developmental delay, the only treatment recommended initially is reassurance and limiting fluids before bedtime. As the child approaches six or seven years of age and problems arise with "sleep-overs," behavior modification usually works well. If enuresis persists, drug therapy is usually successful. The bottom line is that bedwetting is really not usually the child's fault, and he or she should not be blamed or made to feel bad for this problem. Bedwetting will usually resolve spontaneously if given time. Frustrated parents who are tired of changing wet sheets, should just remember that "This, too, will pass."

References

1. Gillenwater JY, Grayhack JT, Howards SS, Duckett JW (eds.): *Adult and Pediatric Urology*, 3rd ed. St. Louis: Mosby, 1996.
2. Macfarlane MT: *Urology for the House Officer*. Baltimore: Williams and Wilkins, 1988.
3. Walsh PC, Retik AB, Stamey TA, Vaughan ED (eds.): *Campbell's Urology*, 6th ed. Philadelphia: W.B. Saunders, 1992.

CHAPTER 3

TORSION

The testicle receives its blood supply via the spermatic cord (Figure 3.1). Torsion occurs when the testicle and spermatic cord twist around a vertical axis, as seen in Figure 3.2. This situation results in venous obstruction, progressive swelling, compromised arterial blood supply, and, if not corrected quickly, death of the testicle.

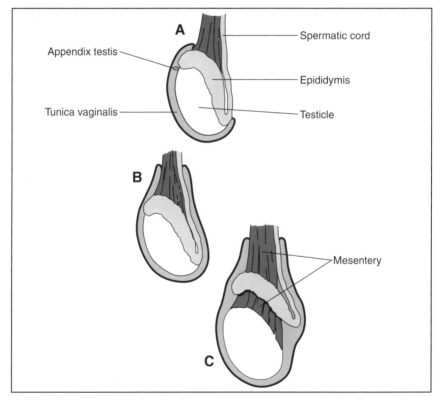

Figure 3-1: *A. Normal anatomy of the scrotum and its contents. The tunica vaginalis does not envelop the epididymis. B. Bell-clapper deformity. The tunica vaginalis envelops the epididymis allowing the testis and cord to rotate within. C. Testis suspended from epididymis, allowing twist to occur between testis and epididymis.*

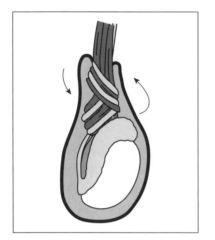

Figure 3-2: Testicular torsion.

Torsion can occur at any age, but it is most common in boys from 12 to 18 years of age. Its cause is unknown; however, it is believed that a narrow mesenteric attachment from the spermatic cord onto the testis is a predisposing factor (Figure 3.1). This narrow attachment allows the testicle to fall forward, making it easier for the testicle to rotate freely within the scrotum, like a clapper in a bell. It has been suggested that contraction of the muscle fibers around the spermatic cord during trauma, exercise, sexual excitement, or exposure to cold exerts a rotary force on the testicle resulting in torsion.

The anatomic abnormality that predisposes to torsion is usually bilateral, meaning it happens on both the left and right sides of the body. For this reason, when torsion is found to exist at operation, the other testis must also be fixed to the scrotum to try to prevent the same situation from occurring on the other side.

The typical patient presents with a sudden onset of testicular pain and swelling, often associated with some minor trauma. Approximately 30 percent of patients report a prior episode of similar pain which resolved spontaneously. Abdominal pain, nausea, and vomiting may occur. This presentation may be confused with a stomach virus, which may result in a delay in seeking medical attention.

The testicle will usually be tender, may be located higher in the scrotum (due to shortening of the twisted cord), and the epididymis may have an anterior location (as opposed to its normal posterior orientation). The *cremaster reflex* (an upward movement of the testicle which usually occurs when the inner aspect of the upper thigh is stroked) is usually absent in patients with torsion.

If any doubt exists as to the possibility of torsion, there are some radiologic tests which may aid in diagnosis. Two of these tests include ultrasound of the scrotum with color flow Doppler to see if blood flow to the testicle exists, and nuclear medicine testicular scan, also to attempt to document the presence or absence of blood flow to the testicle. In torsion, no blood flow to the testis will be seen. If the diagnosis of torsion is strongly suspected, immediate treatment is indicated.

There are other conditions which may cause testicular pain and, thus, may be confused with torsion. Epididymitis (infection or inflammation of the epididymis) is the condition most commonly confused with torsion.

Early on, history and physical examination can usually distinguish the two conditions. However, delayed presentations, with resultant swelling, may make it difficult to differentiate epididymitis from torsion. Other conditions which can cause acute scrotal pain include torsion of a testicular appendage, trauma and, rarely, testicular cancer.

The treatment of testicular torsion consists of immediate detorsion (i.e., untwisting of the spermatic cord to re-establish blood flow to the testicle). Testicular salvage rates depend on the duration of ischemia (lack of blood supply). Approximate salvage rates compared to the duration of torsion are seen below:

Duration of Torsion (hrs)	Testicular Salvage (%)
0-6	85-97
6-12	55-85
12-24	20-55
> 24	<10

Manual detorsion can be attempted by rotating the affected testicle from the midline outward. However, definitive treatment involves surgical exploration, detorsion, and fixation of the testicle to the scrotal wall to prevent recurrence. The obviously unsalvageable testicle is usually removed to prevent complications resulting from a dead testicle (such as wound separation, infection, or possible problems with fertility). In cases of torsion, the opposite testicle also needs to be fixed to the scrotal wall because of the high incidence (up to 42 percent) of its subsequent torsion.

There have been studies suggesting that patients with torsion have decreased fertility, and it appears that the duration of torsion before treatment may affect semen parameters. It has also been suggested that in patients with torsion the fertility capabilities of the other testis may be affected by some, as yet unknown, immune mechanism.

The bottom line is that what goes around does not always come back around. . . Pain in the testicle needs to be evaluated quickly by a qualified physician to make sure that torsion is not missed. Any delay in diagnosing torsion can result in loss of the affected testicle, and may have a deleterious effect on the patient's future fertility.

References

1. Gillenwater JY, Grayhack JT, Howards SS, Duckett JW (eds.): *Adult and Pediatric Urology*, 3rd ed. St. Louis: Mosby, 1996.
2. Macfarlane MT: *Urology for the House Officer*, 2nd ed. Baltimore: Williams and Wilkins, 1995.
3. Smith-Harrison LI and Koontz WW, Jr.: "Torsion of the Testis: Changing Concepts." *AUA Update Series* 1990; vol. 9, lesson 32.
4. Walsh PC, Retik AB, Stamey TA, Vaughan ED (eds.): *Campbell's Urology*, 6th ed. Philadelphia: W.B. Saunders, 1992.

CHAPTER 4

THE SEXUAL ACT

Puberty has been defined as the period in life, usually occurring sometime between the ages of ten and fourteen, during which the reproductive organs mature and reproduction becomes possible. In the male, the testes begin to produce sperm; the genital glands and penis enlarge and become functional; the secondary sex characteristics (e.g., hair pattern and body contour) develop; and the sexual drive is initiated. All of these phenomena are effects of the hormone testosterone, and puberty in the male is due to the onset of increased testosterone secretion by the testes. For those experiencing it, puberty seems much more complicated than this. However, it is during this time that men become extremely aware of the sexual act. This chapter describes the normal physiology of the sexual act. Subsequent chapters will deal with problems that may occur with it.

There are four parts to the male sexual act: erection, emission, ejaculation, and orgasm. (There used to be five parts, but reaching for the remote control is no longer considered to be a true part of the sexual act.) Each of these parts depend on the integration of separate neurologic, hormonal, and hemodynamic mechanisms.

ERECTION

Figure 4.1 depicts the anatomy of the male reproductive system. Penile erectile tissue is contained within three corporeal bodies: two dorsally positioned corpora cavernosa, and a ventrally positioned corpus spongiosum, which also contains the urethra. The ability to have an erection depends on: 1) an intact brain and fully functional nerves; 2) normal blood vessels; 3) adequate hormonal function; and 4) appropriate psychologic input.

Erotic stimulation, triggered by the five senses or by memory, begins the process. The nervous system responds by sending chemical messages

15

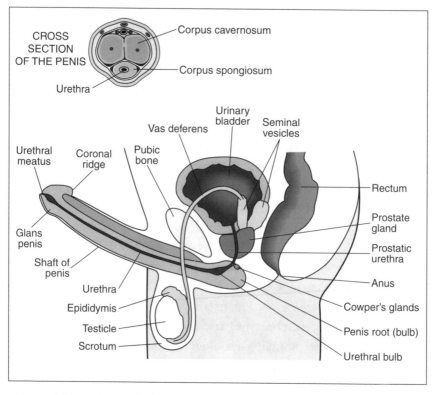

Figure 4-1: *The male reproductive system.*

to and from the pelvic area. This results in increased arterial blood flow to the penis. The smooth muscle tissue in the penis relaxes, allowing more blood to flow into the corpora cavernosa. These corpora fill with blood, resulting in increased size and length of the penis. When all of the vascular spaces of the penis are filled with blood, the organ becomes rigid. It is believed that in the erect state, the filling of the vascular spaces of the corpora cavernosa exerts a strong pressure against the penile veins, greatly reducing their outflow of blood. This increased arterial inflow with decreased venous outflow results in an erection. As long as sexual stimulation is continued, an erect state can normally be maintained until ejaculation and orgasm. Although most physicians would agree that a relationship between male hormones and erectile activity exists, the nature of this relationship and the mechanisms responsible for hormonal control of sexual activity are unclear.

"Reflex" erections may occur through the local reflex arc at the sacral levels of the spinal cord. An example of this occurs when tactile stimulation of the genitalia results in an erection. This explains how approximately 95 percent of patients with upper spinal cord injuries continue to have erections.

EMISSION

Usually, following initiation of erection, sensory nerve impulses from the glans penis reach the spinal cord. The nervous system output causes secretions from the prostate, seminal vesicles, and periurethral glands to be deposited in the prostatic urethra. In addition, sperm from the vas deferens, and probably the tail, or lower part, of the epididymis, are propelled into the prostatic urethra. This part of the sexual act is usually perceived as a pleasant, sometimes itchy, feeling deep inside the urethra and penis, just before ejaculation.

EJACULATION

Distension of the posterior urethra by seminal fluid during emission is believed to trigger specific neural pathways that result in ejaculation. At the time of ejaculation, the bladder neck closes (so that sperm cannot enter the bladder). The external urethral sphincter relaxes, and certain pelvic muscles (the bulbocavernosus and ischiocavernosus muscles) contract spasmodically, expelling semen from the posterior urethra out through the urethral meatus. The fluids secreted by the prostate and seminal vesicles serve as nutrients and a vehicle of transport for the sperm. Once ejaculation has occurred, there is a rapid onset of muscular and psychological relaxation, and an increase in heart rate and blood pressure. There is also a latent period after ejaculation during which a second erection is not possible. This latent period (or refractory period) is variable and may last hours even in perfectly healthy men. It is also age dependent; that is, it generally increases with age.

The average volume of fluid ejaculated is approximately 3 ml, and contains approximately 300 million sperm. However, the range of normal seminal values is wide and will be discussed further in another chapter.

ORGASM

Orgasm is the intensely pleasurable sensation at the end of the sexual act, usually associated with ejaculation. It is primarily a psychologic phenomenon that results from the integration of the other parts of the sexual act with the mind. It is an interesting, though unfortunate, fact of life that men can have only one orgasm per sexual act, whereas women are capable of multiple orgasms during each sexual act.

There are two other topics associated with the sexual act: 1) nocturnal erections; and 2) nocturnal emissions. Erections during sleep were reported in the literature as early as 1940, although they have probably been taking place since Adam's first nap. It has been noted that nocturnal erections, also called nocturnal penile tumescence (NPT), are closely associated with rapid eye movement (REM) sleep. NPT associated with REM sleep is most frequent in pubertal males, occurring five or more times nightly, and steadily declines in frequency and duration with age.

The erection noted on awakening in the morning is believed to have a different etiology. At night as the bladder fills with urine, it can cause a mild obstruction of the venous outflow from the penis, which results in blood accumulation in the penis —the classic "pee hard-on." Once the bladder empties with urination, the erection resolves.

The first time I ever had a "wet dream" (or nocturnal emission, as we say in medicine), I thought that I had wet the bed. When I nervously told my older brother about how I had started to wet the bed again, he reassured me that what was happening was a normal part of life. Nocturnal emissions are, basically, the sexual act occurring during sleep, usually associated with erotic dreams. They are most frequent in pubertal males and decrease in frequency with aging. I'm not sure of the reason behind nocturnal emissions; however, they may be nature's way of "priming the system."

References

1. Gillenwater JY, Grayhack JT, Howards SS, Duckett JW (eds.): *Adult and Pediatric Urology*, 3rd ed. St. Louis: Mosby, 1996.

2. Osbon Medical Systems: *A Patient's Guide for the Treatment of Impotence*. Augusta, Georgia: Charter Publishing Co., 1995.

3. Tanagho EA and McAninch JW (eds.): *Smith's General Urology*, 12th ed. Norwalk, CT: Appleton and Lange, 1988.

4. Vander AJ, Sherman JH, Luciano DS (eds.): *Human Physiology: The Mechanisms of Body Function*, 3rd ed. New York: McGraw-Hill, 1980.

CHAPTER 5

PREMATURE EJACULATION

This chapter, like its topic, will be short and to the point. Premature ejaculation is believed to be the most prevalent form of male sexual dysfunction, affecting an estimated 30 percent of American males. Generally, it is defined as uncontrolled ejaculation with minimal sexual stimulation that occurs before the person wishes to achieve orgasm, sometimes before vaginal penetration, or even before a full erection is reached. The bottom line is that you ejaculate before you want to, or before your partner wants you to, theoretically giving everyone less pleasure.

More recent studies have tried to define premature ejaculation in more objective terms, such as the duration of intravaginal contact (latency time) or the number of thrusts before ejaculation. It appears that in the majority of patients with this problem, the latency time is usually less than two minutes, and orgasm tends to occur with fewer than ten pelvic thrusts. Patients with premature ejaculation can also be subdivided into two groups: primary and secondary. Primary premature ejaculation is that present from the beginning of sexual function, and secondary premature ejaculation occurs after years of "normal" sexual function.

Since ejaculation latency is affected by psychological or cognitive mechanisms, in most cases the cause of premature ejaculation is believed to be psychological. However, since ejaculation is mediated partly through a neural reflex stimulated by sensory input to the penis, a few organic causes of premature ejaculation have also been postulated. Low levels of serum testosterone have been proposed to contribute to this problem, but few studies support this theory. Some investigators have suggested a neurological basis for premature ejaculation. In a recent study, patients with primary premature ejaculation were shown to have hypersensitivity of the glans penis and penile shaft. It is believed that this increased sensitivity predisposes these patients to a shorter latency time. This is an important finding since it may offer an additional approach to the treatment of premature ejaculation.

The goal of treatment is to prolong the time to ejaculation (i.e., the latency time). Some men don't really care about lengthening their latency time. They just want to get their partners to orgasm. In these cases, simple modifications of foreplay techniques may suffice. For example, these men may try to stimulate their partners first, possibly with the use of hand or oral techniques, or even with a vibrator, and then, when their partner is close to orgasm, they may proceed with vaginal intromission or other sexual acts. However, for those wishing to prolong their latency time, there are two basic treatment options: behavior therapy and drugs.

Behavior therapy, or sensate focussing, is based on the theory that it is possible to learn to control your latency time. Years ago, urologists would tell patients to concentrate on other things during intercourse, e.g., the classic, "Think about baseball." However, this worked neither well nor consistently. Some approaches for developing ejaculatory control stem from the work of Dr. James Semans in the 1950's, whose stop-start technique is believed to be the foundation of many of the successful exercises used by sex therapists today. As behavior therapy has become more complex, it has also become more successful in helping men deal with premature ejaculation.

There are many exercises for developing better ejaculatory control, and some of the books listed at the end of this chapter can be very helpful in this regard. The basic programs try to get the patient to learn two skills. One is the ability to attend more fully to their own sensations of arousal and tension, so that they will be able to sense when they are nearing the "point of no return." The other is the ability to make changes in their behavior that will prevent or delay ejaculation. According to a number of studies, approximately 80 percent of men can learn better control in therapy, provided that they are willing to devote the necessary time and energy, especially since it may take up to 20 weeks or more. For persons who do not progress as much as they want by following the programs in these various books, or for those who don't feel comfortable starting with books, an option is to see a qualified sex therapist.

The reported success of drug therapy in premature ejaculation has taken attention away from behavior therapy. The theory behind pharmacotherapy is that various drugs, by affecting the neurologic part of the ejaculatory reflex, or by decreasing anxiety or penile sensation, may increase the latency time and lead to better ejaculatory control.

Clomipramine (trade name Anafranil), a tricyclic antidepressant, has been shown to effectively increase the ejaculatory latency time from approximately two to eight minutes in men with primary premature ejaculation. A dose of 25 mg. is given 12 to 24 hours before attempted sexual activity. Generally, the drug is well tolerated. Side effects have included dry mouth, fatigue, slight dizziness, nausea, and headache. Some of these have disappeared after decreasing the dose by half. The fact that the drug need not be taken long-term, but can be taken as needed, is an attractive feature of this form of therapy.

Fluoxetine (trade name Prozac) at a dose of up to 40 mg. daily was shown to significantly increase the latency time of intravaginal ejaculation compared to placebo. Reported side effects included nausea, headache, and insomnia.

It should be mentioned that drug therapy does not appear to be effective in patients with both premature ejaculation and erectile dysfunction. Also, although preliminary results with drug therapy are promising, additional studies are needed to confirm these findings.

The discovery that patients with premature ejaculation can have penile hypersensitivity has led to drug therapy aimed at diminishing penile sensitivity. Various articles have discussed the use of a desensitizing cream that increases the sensory threshold of the penis with excellent results. This new approach, if substantiated, adds to the armamentarium for the treatment of a very frustrating problem.

Premature ejaculation is a problem that can usually be dealt with successfully, either with behavior therapy alone, or in combination with drug therapy. In most cases, practice *can* make perfect. . .

References

1. Brauer AP and Brauer BJ: *ESO: How You and Your Lover Can Give Each Other Hours of Extended Sexual Orgasm.* New York: Warner Books, 1983.
2. Haensel SM, *et al.*: "Clomipramine and Sexual Function in Men with Premature Ejaculation and Controls." *J Urol* 1996; 156(4):1310-1315.
3. Kara H, *et al.*: "The Efficacy of Fluoxetine in the Treatment of Premature Ejaculation: A Double-Blind Placebo Controlled Study." *J Urol* 1996; 156(5):1631-1632.
4. Xin ZC, *et al.*: "Penile Sensitivity in Patients with Primary Premature Ejaculation." *J Urol* 1996; 156(3):979-981.
5. Zilbergeld B: *The New Male Sexuality.* New York: Bantam Books, 1992.

CHAPTER 6

IMPOTENCE

"The adolescent penis is the penis at its ultimate power. From here on until the end of life, there is a gradual tapering off. Never again will it be so quick to get hard, so stiff, never again will the orgasms be so explosive and the need for them so insistent. There will also be a loss of independence over time. The adolescent penis needs little or nothing from the outside. It gets hard on its own, without needing physical or other kinds of stimulation. As it ages, it will require more stimulation of various sorts."

B. Zilbergeld, *The New Male Sexuality*,
Bantam Books, 1992

The words above, although depressing, are true. There are certain un-avoidable physiologic changes that occur with aging; however, these should not be confused with erectile dysfunction. I have seen countless patients who initially believed that they were having problems with erections, but who, after learning the normal changes that can occur with aging, realized that they didn't have impotence. . . yet. Some of the normal changes that occur with aging include: 1) mild decrease in penile firmness with erection; 2) prolonged time to full erection; 3) increased need for both tactile and psychological stimulation to achieve erection (e.g., when men are young, they can get an erection just thinking about sexual topics; however, as they get older, they require more physical stimulation to get hard); 4) prolonged refractory period (time between erections); and 5) decreased force and volume of ejaculate. Sometimes, however, the problems with erections go beyond these normal changes, and men cross the line into the realm of impotence.

Impotence, also known as erectile dysfunction, is the inability to achieve or maintain erections adequate for vaginal penetration and sexual satisfaction. It is estimated that approximately 10 to 15 percent of all men will have an impotence problem at some time in their life. The incidence of impotence increases with advancing age. This appears to be associated with the increased frequency of certain disease processes with aging, such as hardening of the arteries (atherosclerosis), high blood pressure (hypertension), and diabetes mellitus.

As discussed in Chapter 4, the ability to have an erection depends on normal neurologic, vascular, hormonal, and psychological mechanisms. Problems in any one of these areas can result in erectile dysfunction. The causes of impotence can be divided into three broad categories: 1) psychogenic; 2) organic (related to a disease in which there is a structural change); and 3) iatrogenic (resulting from physicians or medicine).

Psychogenic causes, such as performance anxiety or depression, were thought to account for the majority of the cases of impotence years ago. Today, however, an organic etiology can usually be found in 50 to 90 percent of patients. Psychological problems are usually believed to occupy a secondary role.

Organic causes can be subdivided further into four areas: 1) vascular; 2) hormonal; 3) neurologic; and 4) end organ failure. Vascular problems are believed to be the most common cause of erectile dysfunction. These problems can be due to either decreased arterial inflow or abnormally increased venous outflow —the so-called "venous leak." Diseases such as atherosclerosis, hypertension, and diabetes mellitus have been associated with an increased risk of impotence. Approximately 60 percent of patients with diabetes mellitus for five years or longer have reported some degree of erectile dysfunction. Tobacco smoking can also adversely affect the vessels to the penis. Abnormal venous drainage of the corpora can contribute to erectile insufficiency. If the smooth muscles in the corpora of the penis do not efficiently relax and allow the cavernous spaces to fill with blood, the efferent veins are not compressed and blood escapes from the corpora. Venous leakage is believed to be one of the causes of impotence in patients with Peyronie's disease, which is discussed later in this chapter. Recently, it has been suggested that, in bicycle riders, the blood vessels that supply the penis can get compressed against the pelvic bone by the weight of the rider on the bike seat, and that repeated trauma to these vessels during bicycle riding can result in erectile dysfunction. Studies are currently underway to determine whether bike riding is a risk factor for impotence.

Neurologic problems can also result in impotence. Diseases of peripheral nerves that have been associated with erectile dysfunction include diabetes mellitus, kidney failure affecting the nervous system, and amyloidosis (a condition in which a wax-like protein builds up in various organs of the body, routinely the liver and kidneys). Patients with problems of the spinal cord, such as spinal cord injuries, spina bifida, herniated discs, tumors, or multiple sclerosis, can also have problems with erections. There is little information available concerning the association of cerebral (brain) lesions and sexual potency. Parkinson's disease and Huntington's chorea may affect libido, but their effect on erectile function is unknown. Temporal lobe epilepsy and strokes have been associated with impotence. Presumably the effect is dependent on the site and severity of the lesions.

Hormonal abnormalities can result in impotence; however, the prevalence of endocrine disorders in a population of impotent men is low. Abnormally low levels of testosterone can result in impotence. Other hormonal problems associated with impotence include elevated prolactin levels, thyroid dysfunction, and chronic renal failure. In end stage renal disease (ESRD), partial impotence has been reported to occur in 30 to 80 percent of patients, and total impotence has been seen in 20 to 50 percent. Of note, after renal (kidney) transplantation, most patients report improvement in erectile function. However, if a second transplant is performed, the incidence of impotence is markedly increased, in part due to vascular problems resulting from multiple surgical procedures involving pelvic vessels.

Diseases involving the penis itself can also lead to erectile dysfunction. Two of these problems, Peyronie's disease and priapism, are discussed in detail at the end of this chapter.

Medications are yet another common cause of sexual dysfunction. Even though many classes of drugs may affect erectile function, the two implicated most often are anti-hypertensives taken for high blood pressure and psychiatric or antidepressant compounds. Substance abuse, such as use of illegal drugs or excessive use of alcohol or cigarettes, can seriously damage the blood vessels and nerves involved in normal erections.

Finally, penile trauma and various types of surgery have been associated with impotence. It is common knowledge that radical prostatectomy for treatment of prostate cancer frequently results in erectile dysfunction. However, by modifying the procedure to preserve nerves and vessels to the penis, the occurrence of impotence after this operation has been reduced. Preservation of potency correlates strongly with the patient's age, i.e., the younger the patient, the greater the chance of success. Transurethral resection of the prostate (TURP or "the roto-rooter job") has been reported to result in erectile dysfunction in approximately 5 percent of patients. The occurrence of impotence after surgery for lower bowel disease appears to be dependent on the age of the patient and the extent of the surgical resection. In patients with vascular disease, the risk of sexual dysfunction after aorto-iliac revascularization has been reported to be 20 to 88 percent.

There are numerous complex studies which can be used to evaluate patients with erectile dysfunction. However, as in most diseases, the history and physical examination can often point to a source of the problem. At the initial visit, the urologist tries to determine whether the major disorder is impotence or if the patient suffers from some other sexual dysfunction, such as premature ejaculation or problems with ejaculation or orgasm. Questions concerning recent life crises such as death, divorce, financial problems, or job loss may be used to search for a psychogenic etiology. If patients can get erections during masturbation, while watching erotic videos, or with other partners, a psychogenic source may also be involved. A search is also made for drugs that may cause impotence, such as anti-hypertensives, psychiatric medications, illegal drugs, tobacco and alcohol. Questions regarding heart disease, diabetes mellitus, evidence of vascular disease, or prior surgery can also disclose a reason for impotence. Patients who lack a desire for intercourse may have a hormonal problem resulting in erectile dysfunction. Examination usually includes peripheral pulses (to search for a vascular problem), neurologic exam, and a general examination of the genitalia with special attention to possible palpable plaques along the shaft of the penis (i.e., Peyronie's disease).

Laboratory tests can verify the diagnosis of disorders suspected after the completion of the history and physical examination. Two tests usually employed include a fasting blood glucose and a free testosterone level.

Approximately 12 percent of impotent patients can be found to have unsuspected diabetes mellitus. In addition, even though abnormally low testosterone levels are usually associated with decreased libido, approximately 15 percent of patients with low testosterone levels will not have changes in libido. Other laboratory tests are not usually obtained unless a certain disease process is suspected from the history and physical.

There are many sophisticated special studies which are not usually conducted unless a surgical correction of impotence is contemplated. Some of these studies include: nocturnal penile tumescence studies; penile duplex Doppler ultrasound (a radiologic study that uses sound waves to study penile blood flow); cavernosography (a dye test involving the penile corpora) to search for venous leaks; and arteriography (a dye test involving blood vessels) to search for a problem with arterial inflow.

The goal of treatment for impotence is to help patients and their partners achieve sexual satisfaction. It is recommended that the patient's sexual partner be involved in the treatment discussions if possible, since a successful sexual life for the couple is more likely under these circumstances. As a general rule, the least invasive treatments should be tried first. The major treatment options include: 1) accepting the loss of vaginal penetration with a rigid penis and using alternative methods of sexual gratification; 2) psychological sex therapy counseling; 3) medical therapy; 4) vacuum constriction devices; 5) penile injection therapy; 6) penile prostheses; and 7) vascular surgery.

ACCEPTING THE LOSS OF VAGINAL PENETRATION

Many patients, after hearing the various options for the treatment of erectile dysfunction, may decide against any "artificial" means to achieve erections or sexual satisfaction. Impotent patients and their partners should be made aware of alternative methods of sexual gratification other than vaginal penetration with a rigid penis. If this option is more attractive to an individual couple, they may consider buying a variety of sex therapy books, or even seek out a qualified sex therapist.

PSYCHOLOGICAL SEX THERAPY COUNSELING

Almost every organically based male erectile dysfunction will have psychological overtones. However, if the patient's impotence is thought to be primarily of psychogenic origin, psychotherapy or evaluation by a qualified sex therapist may be beneficial. For example, in patients with depression and impotence, the treatment of their depression may improve their erectile dysfunction. Also, patients with impotence due to performance anxiety may benefit from sex therapy. Best results with sex therapy tend to occur when there is good partner cooperation and both the patient and his partner attend the counseling sessions. The National Register of Health Service Providers in Psychology could help someone find a psychologist with expertise in this area (contact at telephone (202) 783-7663, or internet address *www.nationalregister.com*).

MEDICAL THERAPY

Patients with abnormally low levels of testosterone and partial erectile dysfunction may respond to testosterone administration. However, only a small percentage of impotent males has this problem and will benefit from this treatment. Dosages vary, but usually 200 mg. of testosterone is injected intramuscularly every two to four weeks for several months. If this regimen improves the patient's problem, the treatment is continued; otherwise, alternative treatment options are discussed. Testosterone can be given orally, but studies have shown it to be less effective than intramuscular injections. In addition, there is an increased risk of liver damage with the oral form. Recently, a testosterone patch has become available (Androderm). This patch allows a more physiological restoration of testosterone levels by eliminating the peaks and troughs of injection therapy and by mimicking the natural cycle of testosterone levels through the day since it is applied twice a day. It has been well tolerated, and the most common side effect is transient skin irritation. Therefore, it is recommended that the site of patch placement be rotated.

Although testosterone administration has not been shown to cause prostate cancer, testosterone therapy can speed the growth of a prostate cancer that's already present. As a result, it is important that patients have their prostates evaluated with a digital rectal examination (DRE) and a serum prostate specific antigen level (PSA) before starting testosterone treatments and every six months thereafter, particularly when the patient is over 40 years of age.

Yohimbine is an oral medication that is derived from the bark of the African yohimbine tree. The drug has been used to stimulate desire and improve the quality of erections. A dose of 5 or 5.4 mg. is taken three times a day for one month to test its effect. It costs about $40 per month. Side effects may include headaches, sweaty palms, nervousness, dizziness, and nausea. Although it is usually well tolerated, yohimbine is effective in only a minority of patients, particularly those with psychogenic impotence. Its true effectiveness in double-blind studies is similar to that of a placebo.

Trazodone (Desyrel) is an antidepressant which can cause priapism (abnormally prolonged penile erections) as one of its possible side effects. Due to this well-recognized phenomenon, some investigators have suggested the use of this medication as a potential oral drug for the treatment of impotence. A dose of 50 mg. three times a day resulted in a 65 percent response rate over placebo in a carefully selected patient population. It should be noted, however, that patients with any organic basis for erectile dysfunction were excluded from this study. The major side effect reported was sedation, but it did not usually cause cessation of therapy. Although the use of trazodone has shown some promise, it has not been proven to be effective in follow-up studies and therefore its use in the treatment of impotence should be considered experimental at this time.

Sildenafil (trade name Viagra) is an oral agent which appears to result in relaxation of smooth muscle in the corpora cavernosa. It is this corporeal relaxation that is one of the major events in penile erection. Approximately one hour after ingestion, corporeal relaxation occurs, resulting in spontaneous erection. This drug has been shown to be effective for the treatment of impotence in trials in the United Kingdom and Europe, and became available in the United States in April, 1998. This oral agent comes in doses of 25, 50 or 100 mg., with the usual starting dose being 50 mg. taken approximately 30 minutes to one hour before sexual activity.

The average cost of Viagra is about $9.00 to $10.25 per pill. Initial test results have reported success rates as high as 70 percent. Minimal side effects have been reported, and some of these include mild headache (16 percent), flushing (10 percent), gastric upset (7 percent), nasal congestion (4 percent), temporary visual changes (3 percent), diarrhea (3 percent), dizziness (2 percent), and rash (2 percent).

At present, the only contraindication to the use of Viagra is patients who take nitrates such as nitroglycerin, Nitro-Dur and Nitrostat for heart disease. Long-term studies with Viagra have not yet been concluded. Viagra is discussed in more detail in the next chapter.

Phentolamine (trade name Vasomax), produced by Zonagen, Inc., is also an oral agent which is currently being evaluated for the treatment of impotence. As with Viagra, the use of phentolamine requires sexual stimulation to achieve the desired effect. Initial results in patients with mild degrees of erectile dysfunction have been promising (i.e., approximately 30 percent success rates) with minimal side effects. In addition, there have been no blood pressure changes reported with the use of phentolamine and, therefore, it has no contraindications to use in patients taking nitrates. As a result, oral phentolamine may be an option for impotent patients unable to take Viagra. At present, oral phentolamine is not available, but further studies are in progress to help determine its efficacy and possible place in the treatment of impotence.

Apomorphine is another oral agent being investigated by TAP Pharmaceuticals for the treatment of impotence. It is taken sublingually, which means that it is absorbed by the body after being placed under the tongue rather than being swallowed. Initial clinical trials with apomorphine have reported response rates of up to 50 to 60 percent, with the most common adverse side effect being nausea in 10 to 20 percent of patients. Apomorphine is currently being evaluated for its safety and efficacy, and may become available for use in the United States sometime in 1999.

It should be mentioned that since the various oral agents have different mechanisms of action, there exists the potential for combination therapy as well. That means using two different oral medications at the same time in an attempt to improve the overall effect while requiring lower doses of each agent and possibly decreasing the incidence of adverse side effects. On the same note, combination therapy could also involve using an oral agent with some of the other treatment options available for impotence. It must be stressed, however, that even though combination therapy is a nice idea in theory, the consequences of combination therapy have not yet been determined. Therefore, at present, combination therapy must be considered experimental and cannot be offered, except in properly conducted experimental protocols, until the various combinations have been evaluated in adequate clinical trials.

VACUUM CONSTRICTION DEVICES

Almost every patient who suffers from erectile dysfunction will be a candidate for a vacuum device. There are several similar devices on the market. The typical device consists of a plastic cylinder that fits over the penis. The patient then repeatedly presses a lever that creates a vacuum by pumping air out of the cylinder. This vacuum effect draws blood into the penis, resulting in an erection. The cylinder is removed after a specially-designed rubber tension ring is placed onto the base of the penis to keep blood in the penis and keep it erect during sex. The constriction band should not be kept in place longer than 30 minutes.

The vacuum erection device has been shown to have an excellent patient and partner satisfaction rate. However, some problems may be encountered with this form of therapy. Approximately 40 percent of patients complain of initial discomfort which tends to resolve over time. Small red spots in the skin of the penis (petechiae) due to subcutaneous bleeding has been reported in approximately 25 percent of patients. This can progress to large black and blue areas (ecchymosis) in up to 12 percent of patients. Some users complain that their erections are not as rigid as they want and are somewhat wobbly at the base; however, this is due to the fact that the erection is limited to the penis beyond the constriction band. The penis may also become slightly cold and bluish in color due to the lack of new blood flowing into the penis while the tension ring is in place. Some patients dislike the lack of spontaneity associated with these devices which can be a significant problem for single patients without a steady partner. Uncircumcised patients with tight foreskins may develop significant pain and swelling with the vacuum device, and therefore, may require a circumcision before satisfactory use of the device. Impotent patients with severe penile curvature due to Peyronie's disease may be unable to use the device. Patients on anticoagulants (blood thinners) may be more prone to subcutaneous penile bleeding, and therefore, it is recommended that patients on Coumadin keep the constriction ring on for no more than 15 minutes at a time.

The devices usually cost between $150 and $500, and some of the major manufacturers of these devices have a return policy for the patient who is not satisfied with this form of therapy. As stated earlier, satisfaction has generally been high in patients who have chosen these devices.

PENILE INJECTION THERAPY

Various chemicals, when injected into the corpora cavernosa of the penis, result in cavernosal smooth muscle relaxation, increased penile blood flow, and a subsequent erection. Typically, the urologist will perform these injections in the office until the appropriate dose for each patient is determined. Then, once the patient demonstrates the ability to perform self-injection with good sterile technique, he is given prescriptions for home use.

Papaverine hydrochloride was the first agent widely used for intracavernosal self-injection. It is not approved by the Food and Drug Administration (FDA) for use in the treatment of impotence. Therefore, it is not typically easy to find in outpatient settings.

Prostaglandin E-1 (also known as alprostadil, Caverject, or Prostin VR) has recently been approved by the FDA for intracavernosal injection. Other drugs have been tried as well, and various combinations of these products have also been used to reduce the effective dose of each component needed in an attempt to decrease the side effects from each agent while still achieving an erection. Prostaglandin as a single agent is more effective than papaverine, but costs much more.

Various side effects have been reported with injection therapy. Penile pain with the onset of erection, often of a moderate to severe nature, has been seen, especially with prostaglandin E-1. Since these agents may be absorbed into the circulation, systemic side effects can sometimes be seen. These include dizziness, hypotension (low blood pressure), and headache. The use of a tourniquet at the base of the penis for a few minutes following injection may lessen the incidence of these systemic effects. The presence of significant cardiovascular disease is a relative contraindication for the use of injection therapy since transient hypotension may precipitate an unwelcome event, such as a heart attack or stroke. Also, patients with poor eyesight or poor manual dexterity, or patients with a penile prosthesis in place, are not candidates for this form of therapy. Anatomic deformities of the penis, such as Peyronie's disease, may get worse with continued injection therapy. Finally, patients with a bleeding disorder, or those on Coumadin, are not really candidates for intracavernosal injections due to the increased risk of bleeding.

If the minimum effective dose of intracorporal injection is used, the average duration of an erection should be 30 minutes to an hour. Priapism has been reported in 1 to 18 percent of patients using injection therapy, with an average of 3 percent. This problem requires emergency treatment. Therefore, the patients who choose injection therapy for the treatment of impotence are usually told to seek immediate medical attention if their erections last longer than four hours.

Injection therapy tends to work best in patients with neurogenic or psychogenic impotence, but has been shown to be effective in cases of mild arterial insufficiency. It is much less effective in patients with erectile dysfunction due to venous leaks. There are several medication delivery systems for penile injections that help to reduce anxiety over self-injection by concealing the needle. These devices have several other advantages: 1) patients can penetrate their skin at the touch of a button; 2) the device protects the needle from contamination; and 3) the needle is automatically inserted into the penis to the proper depth each time. The cost of injection therapy varies depending on the drug, or mix of drugs, used. Each injection may cost between $5 and $20, and since it is not recommended to use these injections more often than every other day, the annual cost for injection therapy will usually range from $500 to $2000.

Numerous medications have been tried in the form of topical or intraurethral therapy, mostly without a great deal of success. Recently, Muse has been shown to produce partial to complete erections in approximately 70 percent of patients with minimal side effects. This drug is basically alprostadil in suppository form that is introduced into the urethra, thus eliminating the need for penile injections. The drug has been approved for clinical use by the Food and Drug Administration and was released in the United States in early 1997 by Vivus Inc. After insertion into the urethra, the drug is absorbed into the penis and causes dilation of blood vessels in the penis with increased blood flow. An erection usually begins about five to ten minutes after dosing. Alprostadil is one of the drugs used in injection therapy; however, the suppository form obviates the need for needle injection making this form of therapy more comfortable for the patient. Muse comes in various dosages (125, 250, 500, and 1000 mcg.), but most patients end up using either 500 or 1000 mcg. It is recommended that the drug be stored in a refrigerator but be allowed to warm to room temperature for about 30 minutes prior to insertion. The initial studies reported a 65 percent success rate with Muse, but my experience has been fifty-fifty; that is, about 50 percent of my patients who try Muse are satisfied enough with the results to keep using it. And always remember, something is better than nothing. Muse should not be used more often than once a day.

The most common side effects associated with Muse include temporary aching in the penis, testicles, or perineum (area between the penis and anus); warmth or burning sensation in the urethra; penile redness due to increased blood flow; and minor urethral blood spotting due to improper administration. Other less frequent side effects include prolonged erection and decreased blood pressure, which can result in light-headedness or dizziness (3.0 percent), fainting (0.4 percent), urethral infection, rapid pulse, or swelling of leg veins. Most of the patients I have treated with Muse have tolerated it very well, and no one has reported significant side effects so far.

PENILE PROSTHESIS

The concept of inserting a rigid rod inside the penis to facilitate coitus was an extension of the fact that various animals --for example, dogs, bears, raccoons, and walruses–have a bone called the *os penis* in their penis. Modern penile prostheses consist of two major types of devices: semi-rigid and inflatable. The semi-rigid ones are usually solid silicone cylinders with some type of metallic core or a cable-connected interlocking plastic component system covered by a synthetic sheath. There are three types of inflatable devices: 1) self-contained; 2) two-piece with a combination scrotal pump and reservoir; and 3) three-piece systems with separate scrotal pump and a reservoir that is placed in the lower abdomen. Semi-rigid prostheses have less tendency for mechanical failure, but the flaccidity, concealability, and girth are not optimal. The three-piece devices offer the best flaccidity for concealment, rigidity, and girth, but also require more extensive surgery and have a greater risk of mechanical failure.

Complications of penile prostheses include infection (2 to 7 percent) which usually necessitates removal of the prostheses; erosion of the cylinders through the urethra or the penile shaft (1 to 11 percent); malfunction (up to 40 percent); penile pain, especially in diabetic patients; and penile shortening. Although particle shedding and migration from silicone prosthetic devices has been described, no systemic silicone-induced disorder from a penile prosthesis has been reported.

It is imperative that patients considering a penile prosthesis be fully aware of the possibility of reoperation, which now ranges from 5 to 10 percent. Some patients are dissatisfied with the results of penile prosthesis surgery, and in many cases, this may be due to unrealistic expectations. The "erection" produced by an implant is by no means the same as a previous natural erection. It tends to be smaller, both in length and circumference. The head of the penis is also softer than during a normal, natural erection. At its best, a penile prosthesis makes patients hard enough for vaginal penetration and intercourse; however, patients need to understand that what they get may not look like what they had when they were achieving normal, natural erections. The cost of an implant varies depending on the type of device but it is generally between $6,000 and $15,000, with the inflatable ones being more expensive.

VASCULAR SURGERY

Vascular surgery for impotence is performed for two possible reasons: to repair or bypass clogged or damaged arteries; or to attempt to seal venous leaks. Only a limited number of men are candidates for penile revascularization procedures. The best candidates for arterial surgery are young men whose blood-flow problems stem from trauma such as accidents, and who have no other contributing factors (e.g., atherosclerosis or diabetes mellitus). Even in these highly selected individuals, the success rate of arterial surgery is approximately 50 percent at best.

Surgery for venous leaks has been performed since the early 1980s. Initial success rates were approximately 80 percent; however, longer follow-up has shown that the problem tends to recur. Success rates now reported are closer to 50 percent.

In general, these surgical procedures are still considered investigational, and it is recommended that they be performed only in a research setting with long-term follow-up available.

RELATED DISEASE PROCESSES

There are two disease processes associated with impotence that warrant discussion here: Peyronie's disease and priapism.

Peyronie's Disease

Peyronie's disease is a local inflammatory reaction of unknown etiology which results in fibrosis and plaque formation in the tunica albuginea, or outer-covering, of the corpora cavernosa. Some believe that its underlying cause is local trauma, but others believe it may be an autoimmune phenomenon. Patients may present with a palpable plaque on the shaft of the penis, a bending deformity on erection, painful erection, or erectile dysfunction believed to be due to venous leaks. Since spontaneous resolution can be expected in up to 50 percent of patients, conservative management is recommended initially.

The treatment of Peyronie's disease can be either medical or surgical, and medical therapy is usually prescribed first to allow ample time for spontaneous resolution. Also, because Peyronie's disease can change dramatically in the first 12 months after onset, conservative therapy until plaque stabilization occurs is essential to select the appropriate long-term treatment. Patients with minimal-to-moderate curvature, no penile pain, and continued normal sexual activity require no invasive diagnostic procedures or treatment. If the patient's problem progresses, more aggressive treatments may be indicated.

Oral medications have been used to try to affect plaque formation. Among these, the two used most commonly are vitamin E and para-aminobenzoate potassium (Potaba). No satisfactory studies evaluating any of these agents have been conducted. However, they are well-tolerated and anecdotal reports of success suggest that these medications may be helpful for some patients.

The injection of palpable plaques in an attempt to make these areas of scar tissue more pliable has been studied. Various agents, such as steroids and collagenase, have been tried, but no statistically significant improvement in penile curvature following injection has been reported. Before intralesional injection therapy can be recommended widely, more long-term studies must be conducted.

Significant improvement in penile pain has been described with radiation therapy for Peyronie's disease. Radiation therapy does not improve curvature, plaque size, or erectile function, and since pain is the symptom that most often resolves spontaneously, questions regarding the true efficacy of radiation therapy have arisen.

Surgical treatment of Peyronie's disease should be reserved for those patients with severe deformities precluding penetration and/or sexual activity. Surgical candidates must have stable disease after approximately 12 months from the onset of plaque formation and curvature without evidence of progression. If these patients continue to complain of penile curvature preventing sexual intercourse, inadequate penile rigidity, or other deformities despite medical treatment, surgical intervention may become the only treatment option.

The key point here is that the only reason for surgical intervention is to allow the patient to become sexually active again. In patients with adequate erections but whose penile curvature precludes penetration, a procedure that attempts to straighten the penis is usually successful. In patients with erectile dysfunction and penile curvature, penile prosthesis placement, with or without plaque incision, appears to be the procedure of choice. In patients with Peyronie's disease whose only complaint is pain with erections, results of surgical therapy have been disappointing. Therefore, in general, surgical therapy is only recommended in Peyronie's disease in an attempt to help the patient achieve sexual intercourse.

Priapism

Priapism is defined as an abnormally prolonged penile erection which generally involves only the corpora cavernosa and not the spongiosum around the urethra. The underlying cause of priapism is obstruction of the venous drainage of the penis. The most common reason for this today is pharmacological, especially drugs used for the intracorporal injection therapy of impotence. Other drugs which can result in priapism include antihypertensives and some drugs used to treat psychiatric diseases. Additional causes of priapism include sickle cell disease or trait, which is the most common cause of priapism in children; leukemia and other cancers; trauma, which can result in hematoma formation with subsequent compression of veins which drain the penis; and idiopathic origins, which means that the cause is unknown.

The diagnosis of priapism is not difficult. Patients present with a persistent erection without sexual desire. Pain and fever may be present along with difficulty voiding. In impotent patients treated with injection therapy, if the erection lasts longer than four hours, emergency treatment is indicated. Patients will often delay seeking medical attention because of embarrassment. However, early treatment is crucial since priapism can result in permanent impotence in up to 50 percent of cases.

The initial treatment of priapism usually involves a trial of penile injection with phenylephrine or some other agent to decrease penile arterial inflow (e.g., epinephrine, dopamine, or metaraminol). Oral agents, such as terbutaline, have been tried, but reports of its efficacy are mixed. If pharmacological therapy fails to result in resolution of priapism, an attempt is made to aspirate old stagnant blood from the penis. If this is without success, various surgical procedures have been described to help shunt blood out of the penis. Definitive treatment of priapism should not be delayed because the risk of permanent impotence increases significantly if therapy is not started within 24 hours.

In summary, erectile dysfunction is a very common problem but fortunately a variety of satisfactory treatment options exist. When considering the different treatment options, each patient needs to decide what he and his partner will be most comfortable with. Most experts recommend that the simple, inexpensive, reversible treatments be tried first, while the more complex, expensive, and irreversible treatments be attempted later, if necessary. This is a good policy to help guide decision-making, since you can always move on to more invasive treatment options if the method you start with doesn't help you achieve your desired goal. Once natural erections are no longer possible, there are ways to help men have sexual intercourse as long as they understand and accept the fact that nothing will be as perfect as a normal, natural erection.

References

1. Carson CC: "Peyronie's Disease: Diagnosis and Management." *Mediguide to Urology* 1996; 9(4):1-8.
2. Gillenwater JY, Grayhack JT, Howards SS, Duckett JW (eds.): *Adult and Pediatric Urology*, 3rd ed. St. Louis: Mosby, 1996.
3. Lewis RW and Barrett DM: "Modern Management of Male Erectile Dysfunction." *AUA Update Series* 1995; vol. 14, lesson 20.
4. Lugg J and Rajfer J: "Drug Therapy for Erectile Dysfunction." *AUA Update Series* 1996; vol. 15, lesson 36.
5. Macfarlane MT: *Urology for the House Officer*, 2nd ed. Baltimore: Williams and Wilkins, 1995.
6. Osbon Medical Systems: *A Patient's Guide for the Treatment of Impotence*. Augusta, Georgia: Charter Publishing Co., 1995.
7. Zilbergeld B: *The New Male Sexuality*. New York: Bantam Books, 1992.

CHAPTER 7

VIAGRA

Not since Eve ate "the apple" has taking something by mouth received so much media attention. It seems that Viagra has given new meaning to the classic physician's phrase, "Take two pills and call me in the morning." Given the intense interest in and attention focused on Viagra, it may be worthwhile to devote some extra time to answer some of the more common questions regarding this medication.

Viagra wasn't developed with sexual activity in mind. Initially designed as a drug to improve blood flow in patients with heart disease, Viagra was subsequently found to have an interesting and very desirable side effect. Patients who took it began to report improvement in their ability to achieve and maintain erections. Since no successful oral agent to treat impotence existed, this remarkable observation led Pfizer, the drug company which developed Viagra, to pursue further studies in this area. The rest is history.

How does Viagra work?

First, a brief review of the process of erection. In response to sexual stimuli (e.g., visual, mental, tactile, or any combination of these), a chemical, known as nitric oxide, is released in the corpus cavernosum of the penis. The presence of nitric oxide stimulates the formation of another chemical called cyclic GMP. Increased levels of cyclic GMP, in some as yet unknown way, result in relaxation of the muscle cells in the corpora cavernosa and increased blood flow to the penis, which leads to erection. An enzyme called cyclic GMP phosphodiesterase type 5 (PDE-5) breaks down cyclic GMP. Lower levels of cyclic GMP results in less penile blood flow and resolution of the erection. Viagra selectively inhibits cyclic GMP PDE-5. By inhibiting the enzyme which breaks down cyclic GMP, Viagra encourages higher levels of cyclic GMP in the penis in response to sexual stimulation. Viagra cannot have any effect in the absence of activation of the nitric oxide/cyclic

GMP pathway. Therefore, Viagra can help produce erections only when sexual stimulation is present. In other words, Viagra doesn't work if "the moment isn't right."

What is the usual dose of Viagra?

Viagra comes in doses of 25, 50, and 100 mg., with the usual starting dose being 50 mg. taken approximately 30 minutes to 1 hour before sexual activity. In patients with liver problems, the recommended starting dose is 25 mg.

How much does Viagra cost?

The cost of one pill may range from $9 to $10.25.

Will Viagra work for me?

Initial test results reported success rates as high as 70 percent. Viagra appears to be effective in the treatment of patients with impotence regardless of severity, underlying cause (i.e., organic, psychogenic, or mixed), race, and age. Even 43 percent of patients with impotence after radical prostatectomy reported improved erections with Viagra.

It is important to stress that, as stated prior, Viagra requires sexual stimulation to exert an effect (you can't just take the pill and expect to get an erection). So, in the absence of sexual stimulation, taking Viagra will probably just give you a headache and red ears. In addition, Viagra does not have any beneficial effect in patients without problems having erections, and should not be used in patients without impotence.

Will I get used to Viagra and note a decreased response to it as time goes on?

Although Viagra has only been around for a short time, greater than 85 percent of patients who initially responded in clinical trials continued to respond on follow-up studies. Therefore, at present, it does not appear that patients develop a tolerance to this drug over time.

What side effects can I expect with Viagra?

The most frequently reported side effects of Viagra include: 1) transient headache (16 percent); 2) flushing (10 percent); 3) mild stomach upset (7 percent); 4) nasal congestion (4 percent); 5) urinary tract infection (3 percent); 6) abnormal vision (3 percent); 7) diarrhea (3 percent); 8) dizziness (2 percent); and 9) rash (2 percent). Most of the side effects were mild and lasted a few minutes to a few hours after dosing, and only 2 percent of patients withdrew from the studies because of treatment-related side effects.

As per the visual disturbances, these usually involved transient changes in the perception of color hue or brightness. Some people have joked that they would rather take Viagra and keep their eyes closed during intercourse to avoid the visual side effects than to not take the pill at all. It must be stressed, however, that the long-term effects of Viagra on vision, and/or any other system of the body, are as yet unknown, and only time will answer these questions completely.

I've heard about people dying from Viagra. Are there any contraindications to its use?

Since Viagra causes dilation of blood vessels, its use in patients taking nitrates can result in significant decreases in blood pressure and even shock or death. Nitrates include drugs such as nitroglycerin, Nitro-Dur, Nitrostat, Transderm Nitro, etc. There are three common scenarios in which Viagra users could suffer significant consequences:

- The patient with heart disease who gets chest pain during intercourse may reach for his nitroglycerin tablet. The combination of Viagra and nitroglycerin could cause a significant drop in blood pressure, known as shock.
- Men without a history of heart problems who experience chest pain during intercourse after having taken Viagra. If the paramedics or emergency room physician are unaware that the patient took Viagra, they may give him a nitroglycerin tablet to try to relieve his chest pain, causing shock.

- The man who takes Viagra and then inhales amyl nitrate (a street drug used to enhance intercourse, also called "poppers") could also go into shock.

As a result of this significant drug interaction, the use of Viagra is contraindicated in patients who take nitrates. Even patients who carry a bottle of nitroglycerin tablets with them just in case they experience an attack of angina should consider other options for the treatment of impotence.

What about the use of Viagra for women?

The theory behind this topic involves studies in women with vaginal engorgement insufficiency syndrome. In this condition, post-menopausal women have problems producing vaginal secretions for adequate lubrication. Even supplemental estrogens (female hormones) do not improve the problem in some women. The lack of adequate lubrication results in painful intercourse, so these women have decreased desire for intercourse due to the fear of it being painful. Viagra does not increase the desire for intercourse; however, the theory is that taking Viagra could increase blood flow in the tissues around the vagina. Increased blood flow with resultant engorgement of the vaginal walls leads to an increase in vaginal secretions. It is believed that this increase in vaginal lubrication would improve the sex act for these women. This theory is in the process of being studied, but at the present time, the only indication for the use of Viagra is in men with erectile dysfunction. So right now, ladies, I'm sorry! On a brighter note, however, K-Y jelly is a lot cheaper than Viagra!

Viagra has still only been around for a relatively short time, and we're learning more about it each day. Also, newer treatment options are constantly being developed. The bottom line is that Viagra is good, but it won't work for everyone. Therefore, it is nice to know that there are other safe and effective alternatives for the treatment of this very common problem.

Reference

1. Goldstein I, *et al.* "Oral Sildenafil in the Treatment of Erectile Dysfunction." *New Engl J Med* 1998; 339(1):59

CHAPTER 8

RETROGRADE EJACULATION

As discussed in Chapter 4, the seminal fluid is deposited into the prostatic urethra via the ejaculatory ducts (emission). After this, the bladder neck closes, and contraction of the bulbocavernosus and ischiocavernosus muscles propels semen out through the urethra. The failure of bladder neck closure to occur simultaneously with contraction of the cavernosal and pelvic floor musculature results in retrograde flow of semen into the bladder.

Retrograde ejaculation is defined as the propulsion of the seminal fluid backwards into the bladder rather than antegrade through the urethra during the ejaculatory process. This situation usually results in a smaller ejaculate volume and, therefore, a smaller wet spot, which may be a relief to some people. However, an unexplained decrease in ejaculate volume can also be very disconcerting to some men. In addition, since urine is usually spermicidal due to its acidic pH, retrograde ejaculation can result in infertility. Retrograde ejaculation is usually not clinically significant, because most of these patients are beyond their reproductive years.

Malfunction of the bladder neck can occur either because of interruption of its nerve supply (pharmacologic or traumatic) or because of damage to the smooth muscle fibers of the bladder neck.

Anatomic abnormalities leading to retrograde ejaculation are usually the result of surgical interventions. Transurethral resection of the prostate (TURP) is one of the most common causes, with an incidence of up to 90 percent, depending on the degree of tissue resected in the area of the bladder neck. Open removal of the prostate (suprapubic or retropubic prostatectomy) or any other surgical procedure that alters the integrity of the bladder neck can result in retrograde ejaculation. Urethral strictures from prior surgery or infections have also been reported to occasionally result in retrograde ejaculation.

Some of the congenital conditions reported to cause retrograde ejaculation include abnormal position of the ejaculatory duct, exstrophy (an abnormality in the development of the bladder which also affects the bladder neck function), and posterior urethral valves (obstructing pieces of tissue in the urethra which can block the antegrade flow of semen resulting in backflow of semen into the bladder).

Any neurologic problem that affects the innervation of the bladder neck muscles can prevent their normal closure during ejaculation. Retroperitoneal lymph node dissection (surgery to remove lymph tissue from the posterior part of the abdomen) in patients with certain testicular cancers can result in retrograde ejaculation. Extensive colorectal or vascular surgery may lead to similar nerve injury. Spinal cord injuries may also affect the nerves to the bladder neck with resultant retrograde ejaculation. Also, diabetes mellitus has also been reported to cause this problem in some patients. These patients often have other findings related to impaired neurologic function.

Various drugs can affect seminal emission and/or ejaculation, which can lead to failure of emission or retrograde ejaculation. The major classes of drugs that may lead to this problem are antihypertensives and psychotropic agents, such as antidepressants or tranquilizers.

Finally, idiopathic retrograde ejaculation (i.e., that without an obvious cause) has been reported. However, the diagnosis of idiopathic retrograde ejaculation should be made only after thorough investigation.

The diagnosis of retrograde ejaculation is often straightforward. The patient may complain of a "dry ejaculate" or a decreased volume of ejaculate, but sometimes the problem will be discovered in the evaluation of infertility. Patients may have a history of prostate or urethral surgery. The presence of sperm on the urinalysis obtained after ejaculation, along with a small ejaculate volume, is diagnostic of this problem.

The treatment of retrograde ejaculation varies depending on the situation. Patients who do not desire any more children require no specific therapy and may even appreciate the smaller wet spot. In men with infertility attributable to retrograde ejaculation, the initial therapeutic approach is usually pharmacologic. Various drugs have been used in an attempt to stimulate closure of the bladder neck and, thus, increase the sperm count of the ejaculate. Some of these agents include ephedrine, pseudoephedrine, dextroamphetamine sulfates, phenylpropanolamine, imipramine, and some antihistamines. Side effects of these drugs can include hypertension and low heart rate. Response to therapy is determined by the return of antegrade ejaculation and the percentage of sperm in the ejaculate as compared to sperm remaining in the bladder. Success rates of correcting retrograde ejaculation pharmacologically may be as high as 40 percent. However, patients with retrograde ejaculation resulting from bladder neck surgery generally do not respond to pharmacologic manipulation.

When drug therapy fails to result in adequate antegrade ejaculation, sperm may be retrieved from the bladder for artificial insemination. Methods to recover sperm from the bladder have included: emptying the bladder via catheterization and mixing this fluid with an appropriate buffered solution to prevent sperm death due to acidic urine; or emptying the bladder both prior to and immediately after ejaculation in order to recover the ejaculated fluid in as small a volume of urine as possible. In rare instances, pregnancy has been reported after having the man void intravaginally immediately following intercourse.

Retrograde ejaculation is commonly seen as a result of prostate surgery, and in this age group it is usually of little clinical significance. It may, however, be a cause of infertility in younger patients. With today's technology, the treatment of retrograde ejaculation in these patients can result in successful pregnancies. And remember, as an old professor of mine once said, "retrograde ejaculation is better than *no* ejaculation."

References

1. Gillenwater JY, Grayhack JT, Howards SS, Duckett JW (eds.): *Adult and Pediatric Urology*, 3rd ed. St. Louis: Mosby, 1996.
2. Kaufman DG and Nagler HM: "Specific Nonsurgical Therapy in Male Infertility." *Urologic Clinics of North America* 14(3): 489-498.

CHAPTER 9

HEMATOSPERMIA

Few things in life are as anxiety-provoking to a man or his partner as the sight of blood in the semen. Blood in the seminal fluid, known as hematospermia or hemospermia, is a common complaint in middle-aged men. Often it is the wife or sexual partner who recognizes the symptom. The appearance of the blood can vary from bright red to a brownish color.

Figure 9.1 depicts the normal anatomy of the male reproductive tract. The sperm travels from the testicles through the vas deferens and into the ejaculatory duct, which passes through the prostate and empties into the prostatic portion of the urethra. The seminal vesicles and the prostate are accessory sex glands that secrete fluid that aids in the ejaculatory process (i.e., it contains nutrients for the sperm, or factors that help to liquefy the semen). Blood in the semen can come from any of the organs through which the ejaculate passes. Therefore, hematospermia usually originates from either the seminal vesicles or the prostate.

Some of the more common causes of hematospermia include: 1) hyperplasia of the lining of the seminal vesicles, which is usually the diagnosis used when no obvious source can be found; 2) seminal vesiculitis (infection or inflammation of the seminal vesicles); 3) prostatitis (infection or inflammation of the prostate); and 4) prostate cancer. This symptom has also been reported in patients with prostatic polyps, tuberculosis, or cysts in the prostatic urethra. Tumors of the seminal vesicles can result in hematospermia, but these are extremely rare. The most common cause of hematospermia today is probably iatrogenic (resulting from physicians or medicine). For example, biopsy of the prostate to evaluate for possible prostate cancer can result in hematospermia for up to several weeks after the biopsy.

The evaluation of hematospermia is aimed at ruling out treatable causes, such as infection or prostate cancer. Patients with seminal vesiculitis

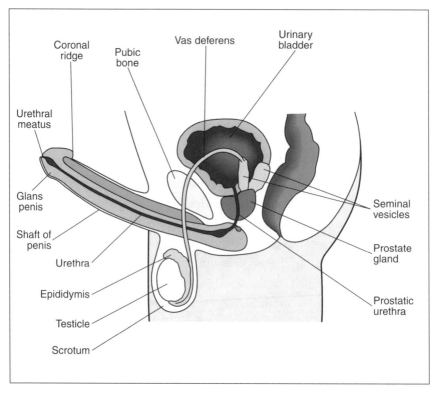

Figure 9-1: *The male reproductive system.*

or prostatitis usually have voiding symptoms, such as burning with urination or frequent voiding. Painful ejaculation may also be seen with these infections. The physical examination may reveal a tender prostate in prostatitis or seminal vesiculitis, and it may reveal a hard, nodular prostate in patients with prostate cancer. A urinalysis and urine culture may point to an inflammatory source. The urinalysis is also important to evaluate for blood in the urine (hematuria) which would require a more in-depth search for a source. Drawing blood for a prostate specific antigen (PSA) test is essential to evaluate for prostate cancer in patients with hematospermia. A thorough urologic investigation of men without other symptoms almost never reveals a pathologic lesion.

The treatment of patients with hematospermia varies depending on clinical suspicion. If the evaluation is consistent with prostatitis or seminal vesiculitis, antibiotic therapy is indicated. If prostate cancer is suspected, further evaluation with a prostate biopsy may be recommended. In patients with significant hematospermia after prostate biopsy, all that is usually necessary is conservative treatment with increased fluid intake and avoidance of blood-thinners —such as aspirin, ibuprofen, or Coumadin— until the bleeding resolves. When there is no evidence to suggest infection, inflammation, prostate cancer, or some other significant lesion, or if the patient has minimal blood-spotting in the semen after prostate biopsy, watchful waiting and reassurance are the treatments of choice.

Hematospermia can be an anxiety-producing symptom. Although medical evaluation is necessary to exclude significant causes, in most cases, hematospermia is of no clinical consequence and just makes the sexual act . . . more colorful.

References

1. Blandy J: *Urology*. Oxford: Blackwell Scientific Publications, 1976.
2. Gillenwater JY, Grayhack JT, Howards SS, Duckett JW (eds.): *Adult and Pediatric Urology*, 3rd ed. St. Louis: Mosby, 1996.
3. Tanagho EA and McAninch JW: *Smith's General Urology*, 12th ed. Norwalk CT: Appleton and Lange, 1988.
4. Walsh PC, Retik AB, Stamey TA, Vaughan ED (eds.): *Campbell's Urology*, 6th ed. Philadelphia: W.B. Saunders, 1992.

CHAPTER 10

VARICOCELE

V aricose veins in the lower extremities can give a person ugly legs. Varicose veins in the scrotum result in a condition which usually feels like a bag full of worms.

A varicocele is an abnormal dilatation of the veins of the spermatic cord. It can be found in up to 20 percent of healthy adolescents and young men, and is rarely detected in boys under ten years of age. It is found more commonly on the left side, with isolated right varicoceles seen in less than 2 percent of males. Bilateral varicoceles can occur in up to 1 percent of males.

Varicoceles are of particular interest because of their association with infertility. They have been detected in up to 40 percent of infertile male patients. Scrotal varicoceles are the most common surgically reversible abnormality found in the subfertile male. However, not all varicoceles require surgical correction. Of all men with varicoceles, only approximately one-third are found to be subfertile.

Various theories have been proposed regarding the cause of varicoceles; however, no single model to explain their genesis is uniformly accepted. Since no other species has been found to have this problem, varicoceles are believed to be a consequence of man's upright posture. It is generally agreed that various anatomic conditions contribute to increased pressures and pooling of blood in the veins of the spermatic cord, resulting in abnormal enlargement and tortuosity of these veins.

Patients with a varicocele may complain of a swelling in the scrotum or may report scrotal discomfort after long periods of standing due to the size of the varicocele. The cornerstone of varicocele diagnosis is an accurate physical examination. Varicoceles can be classified according to size as follows: 1) small (palpable only with straining); 2) moderate (palpable in the standing position without increasing intra-abdominal pressure); and 3) large (visible through the scrotal skin). A variety of diagnostic tests have been used to detect varicoceles not apparent on physical examination (i.e., subclinical varicoceles). However, since the significance of subclinical varicoceles remains controversial, adjunctive diagnostic tests are usually recommended only to confirm the clinical diagnosis or to look for contralateral varicoceles.

Despite intense scientific research, the cause of the testicular dysfunction and resulting infertility in patients with varicoceles remains poorly understood. Some of the mechanisms for infertility that have been proposed include: 1) decreased oxygen delivery to the testicle by venous stasis; 2) retrograde flow of toxins from the renal vein down into the testicular veins; 3) elevation of scrotal temperatures by the blood that pools in the scrotal veins; and 4) depression of hormonal secretion.

Abnormal semen quality in the presence of a varicocele is an indication for repair. Therefore, patients with a clinical varicocele are advised to have a semen analysis to look for abnormalities in semen quality which could result from the varicocele. However, obtaining a semen analysis from an adolescent patient with a varicocele is controversial. Therefore, other criteria that attempt to determine the significance of a varicocele, especially in adolescents, have been devised. Other indications for varicocele repair (varicocelectomy) include: 1) significant size difference (greater than 2 cc.) between the two testicles; 2) progressive decrease in the size of the testicle on the side of the varicocele on follow-up examinations; and 3) bilateral varicoceles in adolescents.

Varicocelectomy has been shown to benefit the infertile male. Between 50 to 80 percent of men who undergo this procedure show improved semen parameters and 23 to 52 percent of patients have been reported to initiate a pregnancy. It has been reported that large varicoceles are associated with greater preoperative impairment of semen quality than smaller varicoceles. However, varicocelectomy of larger varicoceles is associated with greater improvement in semen quality resulting in similar overall pregnancy rates, regardless of the initial size of the varicocele.

Varicoceles can be treated in a variety of ways: 1) open surgical techniques; 2) percutaneous venous occlusion; and 3) laparoscopic techniques.

Surgical varicocelectomy (surgical repair of the varicocele) remains the most popular method of treating varicoceles. The goal is to achieve complete interruption of the venous drainage of the testicles by ligating, or tying off, these dilated veins. Several approaches have been described for the open repair, with success rates ranging from 80 to 100 percent.

When the percutaneous method is employed, radiographic techniques are used to localize the abnormal veins of the spermatic cord. Then, sclerosing agents, metal coils, or both can be used to occlude these abnormal veins. At the present time, most urologists would agree that percutaneous transvenous ablation of varicoceles should be reserved for cases of failed surgical repair.

Laparoscopic varicocelectomy uses a laparoscope, or fiberoptic scope, inserted through the belly-button to guide additional instruments which are placed through smaller ports in the abdomen to ligate the spermatic cord veins. Due to expense, a requirement for general anesthesia, and the small but real potential for major complications, laparoscopy is not presently considered equivalent to open surgery as first-line therapy for varicocele correction.

Not all varicoceles require surgical correction. However, if there is scrotal discomfort secondary to this lesion, if the testis ipsilateral to (i.e., on the same side as) the scrotal varix is found to be atrophic, or if there is reasonable suspicion that impaired semen quality may be related to the presence of the varicocele, surgery should be considered.

References

1. Gillenwater JY, Grayhack JT, Howards SS, Duckett JW (eds.): *Adult and Pediatric Urology*, 3rd ed. St. Louis: Mosby, 1996.
2. Macfarlane MT: *Urology for the House Officer*, 2nd ed. Baltimore: Williams and Wilkins, 1995.
3. Turek PJ and Lipshultz LI: "The Varicocele Controversies I: Etiology and Pathophysiology." *AUA Update Series* 1995; vol. 14, lesson 13.
4. Turek PJ and Lipshultz LI: "The Varicocele Controversies II: Diagnosis and Management." *AUA Update Series* 1995; vol. 14, lesson 14.

5. Wessells H and Van Arsdalen KN: "Surgery of Male Infertility. Part I: Varicocelectomy, Testis Biopsy, and Vasography." *AUA Update Series* 1994; vol. 13, lesson 10.

CHAPTER 11

INFERTILITY

Approximately 85 percent of couples who are practicing unprotected intercourse and seriously trying to achieve a pregnancy will do so within one year. Primary infertility affects only about 15 percent of couples. In this group, about half of the males will demonstrate a significant abnormality that is responsible for, or contributes to, this problem. In order to better understand the evaluation and treatment of male factor infertility, a knowledge of the anatomy and physiologic processes of the male reproductive system is helpful.

The normal adult testes are a pair of ovoid structures usually measuring 4.0 to 5.5 cm. in length, 2.5 cm. in width, and 3.0 cm. in the anteroposterior dimension (from the front to the back). They lie in the scrotum with the long axis upright and tilted slightly forward. The left testis is generally lower than the right. The outer covering of the testicles is a dense, fibrous tissue known as the *tunica albuginea.* The *parenchyma,* or meat, of the testes is composed of tiny convoluted tubules known as the *seminiferous tubules.* Within these tubules, *spermatozoa* are formed and mature. *Sertoli cells,* which are believed to help in the normal development of the sperm, are also located within the seminiferous tubules. Also within the testes, but outside the seminiferous tubules, are located the *Leydig cells* which produce the hormone testosterone. The seminiferous tubules all eventually join to form a network of tubules called the *rete testis,* which is located near the upper part of the testes. These rete testes terminate in 12 to 20 *ductuli efferentes,* which are tubes that carry the sperm from the testicle to the *epididymis.*

The epididymis is a convoluted duct located at the posterolateral aspect of the testicle. It is believed that sperm achieve the ability to fertilize an egg in the epididymis. This is called capacitation. Therefore, the metabolic function of the sperm is greatly enhanced by the epididymis. The epididymis eventually tapers to become the vas deferens which joins with the seminal vesicle to form the ejaculatory duct which, in turn, passes through the prostate and enters the urethra at the level of the prostate.

As stated earlier, the production of sperm (a process called *spermatogenesis*) takes place in the seminiferous tubules in the testes. Spermatogenesis requires normal cells and the appropriate hormonal milieu, especially adequate levels of testosterone produced by the Leydig cells. The production of these hormones is controlled by other hormones which are released from the pituitary gland.

It is believed that in the correct hormonal environment, normal sperm producing cells, known as *germ cells*, continue to divide producing new spermatozoa which move through the seminiferous tubules by a combination of muscle contraction and fluid flow. The sperm then eventually move into the epididymis where they mature and gain the ability to fertilize an egg. Some sperm stay in the epididymis while some move up the vas deferens to be stored in the seminal vesicle until the sexual act. During emission and ejaculation, sperm in the ejaculate comes from both the seminal vesicles and the epididymis.

Even with this brief and superficial overview of male reproductive function, one can see that a lot of complicated processes must go right in order to produce a healthy ejaculate. A review of the common causes of male infertility is seen in Table 11.1

In order to determine the source of infertility, physicians use a complete history, physical examination, and certain laboratory tests. A thorough history is very important in the evaluation since certain events in the patient's past may point to a reason for the problem. It is helpful to know whether or not either partner has ever achieved a pregnancy and if any prior evaluations or treatments have been attempted. A sexual history is usually obtained, including information on any problems with erections, the use of lubricants which may contain spermicides, the timing and the frequency of intercourse. These points are used to determine if the couple's timing of intercourse coincides with the female partner's ovulation to optimize temporal factors.

| Table 11-1: Causes of Male Infertility ||
Diagnosis	%
Varicocele	37.4
Idiopathic (unknown)	25.4
Testicular failure	9.4
Obstruction	6.1
Undescended testes	6.1
Low semen volume	4.7
Agglutination problems	3.1
Sexual dysfunction	2.8
Viscosity problems	1.9
Ejaculatory failure	1.2
Hormonal problems	0.9

Modified from Greenberg SH, *et al.*: "Experience with 425 Subfertile Male Patients." *J Urol* 1978; 119(4):507-510.

Childhood illnesses can also affect fertility. Bilateral or unilateral undescended testicles, regardless of the time of orchiopexy (placing and fixing the testicle in the scrotum), results in poorer semen quality than in patients with normally descended testicles. A history of testicular torsion has been associated with decreased fertility. Mumps after puberty can result in testicular damage with atrophy of the affected testicle in up to 30 percent of patients.

Prior surgery can also have a profound effect on fertility. Hernia repair or scrotal surgery as a child could have led to inadvertent damage to the vas deferens with subsequent obstruction of this tube. Any surgery involving the bladder neck could result in retrograde ejaculation. Testicular cancer has been associated with an infertility rate of approximately 80 percent due to sequelae of chemotherapy, radiation therapy, retroperitoneal surgery, or a combination of all three.

A history of cystic fibrosis can point to obstruction, or absence, of the vas deferens or epididymis. Prior venereal diseases or tuberculosis can lead to scarring and obstruction in the epididymis and/or vas deferens.

In addition, various medications such as nicotine, alcohol, marijuana, sulfasalazine (a medication used to treat inflammatory bowel diseases, such as ulcerative colitis and Crohn's disease), and cimetidine (Tagamet) can affect spermatogenesis. Elimination of these substances may help improve semen quality. Anabolic steroids, such as those taken by some bodybuilders and other athletes, can suppress the normal production of sperm.

Any generalized injury or trauma, such as a fever or virus, can impair testicular function temporarily. Since it takes about 74 days between the formation of new sperm and their appearance in the ejaculate, the effects of an injury can be detected for up to three months after that trauma. Therefore, if a patient gives a history of significant medical problems in the three months prior to the first office visit and if the semen analysis shows abnormal semen quality, the evaluation is usually repeated in another three months before making a decision regarding the quality of sperm production.

The physical examination of the "infertile" male is usually thorough, with emphasis placed on the genitalia. Inadequate virilization, as evidenced by decreased body hair, apparent breast tissue, or decreased penile size, can point to a hormonal abnormality. Abnormal location of the urethral meatus can result in improper placement of the ejaculate within the vaginal vault. Decreased testicular size is also often associated with impaired spermato-genesis. If the epididymis is indurated or nodular, a prior problem which may have resulted in obstruction of the epididymis or vas deferens can be suspected. Engorgement of the veins of the spermatic cord should be searched for, since a varicocele is the most common surgically reversible abnormality found in the subfertile male. A rectal examination is usually performed to search for abnormalities in the prostate or seminal vesicles, which may suggest obstruction of the ejaculatory ducts.

Since an appropriate hormonal environment must exist for the normal function of the reproductive organs, certain laboratory tests can be used to search for hormonal or testicular dysfunction. A preliminary evaluation usually includes assessment of serum levels of luteinizing hormone (LH), follicle-stimulating hormone (FSH), and testosterone. Low levels of FSH or LH, in the presence of low testosterone levels, can point to problem with the pituitary gland. A compensatory rise in FSH levels is usually seen in response to testicular dysfunction. Therefore, in the past, significant eleva-tions in FSH levels in patients with abnormal semen quality usually implied severe testicular failure and, thus, a poor prognosis.

As stated earlier in this chapter, in up to 50 percent of infertile couples there is either a primary male factor or an impaired semen quality sufficient to reduce the probability of pregnancy. Therefore, one of the first tests performed in the evaluation of the infertile couple is usually a semen analysis (the examination of the seminal fluid).

Spermatozoa were first described in the human semen in 1677. However, the difference between normal and abnormal forms was not noted until the 1900s. Since the information obtained from the analysis of the seminal fluid depends on events preceding these examinations, certain standard collection recommendations have been developed. Routinely, 48 to 72 hours of abstinence from sex is suggested before collection of the specimen. Longer periods of abstinence can produce a larger volume of sperm, but they will have poorer motility. Shorter periods of abstinence can result in decreased volumes or decreased number of sperm. The specimen is usually collected in a wide-mouthed container with a screw top, and the patient is told to try to get all of the specimen in the container. Attempts should be made to deliver the specimen to the laboratory within 1.5 hours of collection, and the specimen should be kept as close to body temperature as possible (i.e., kept in a jacket or pants pocket). Usually, a post-ejaculate urine specimen is obtained to exclude retrograde ejaculation. The normal basic semen parameters are seen in Table 11.2.

Table 11-2: Normal Semen Values	
Volume	2.0 ml. or more
pH	7.2 - 7.8
Sperm concentration	20 million sperm/ml. or more
Total sperm count	40 million sperm or more
Motility	50% or more
Morphology (shape)	50% or more with normal morphology
Viability	50% or more live sperm
White blood cells	Fewer than 1 million/ml.

Modified from Gilbert BR, *et al.*: "Semen Analysis in the Evaluation of Male Factor Subfertility." *AUA Update Series* 1992, 11(32):250.

Once the semen analysis is obtained, a review of the results usually yields one of three predominant patterns: 1) normal semen parameters; 2) absence of sperm (azoospermia); or 3) abnormal semen parameters other than azoospermia. Categorizing the results into these three groups usually helps the physician to formulate further diagnostic and treatment plans.

In "infertile" men who present with normal seminal parameters, one of two possibilities exist: their partners have a problem that predisposes the couple to infertility, or these male patients have a problem with sperm function. In the case of normal semen parameters, it is usually recommended that the male's partner undergo a careful evaluation first. If no abnormality is found or if female problems adequately treated do not result in pregnancy, then more sophisticated tests of sperm function can be carried out.

In patients with azoospermia, a post-ejaculate urinalysis is obtained to rule out the possibility of retrograde ejaculation (see Chapter 8). Once retrograde ejaculation is excluded, there are three general possibilities: 1) absence or obstruction of the ducts leading from the testicle to the urethra; b) abnormal testicular function; or 3) hormonal deficiencies. A serum FSH level is usually obtained to help figure out the problem. If the level of FSH is normal or mildly elevated, further studies to search for obstruction, as well as a testicular biopsy to evaluate testis function, are usually performed. Years ago, if the FSH level was greater than three times normal and the testicles were abnormally small, testicular failure was assumed and testis biopsy was not recommended. Couples had to pursue either artificial insemination with another male donor, or adoption. Recently, however, it has been found that approximately 30 percent of male patients with azoospermia and significantly elevated levels of FSH can be shown to have mature sperm on testis biopsy. Since sperm obtained in this fashion could be used for *in vitro* fertilization (IVF), this group of patients should now consider testicular biopsy if IVF is an acceptable approach for the couple.

Nearly 55 percent of all male patients with infertility will demonstrate abnormalities in more than one of the seminal parameters listed in Table 11.2. Again, the FSH measurements can be helpful. If the FSH level is lower than normal, pituitary disease or hormonal deficiencies should be explored. When the FSH level is normal or mildly elevated, a search for exposure to drugs, heat, stress, or environmental toxins is usually made. It should be emphasized that the most common cause of an abnormal semen analysis is a scrotal varicocele (see Chapter 10).

Isolated abnormal seminal parameters occur in 37 percent of men with infertility. In patients with low semen volumes (less than 2 ml.), some possibilities include: 1) collection error (such as not getting all of the specimen in the container); 2) retrograde ejaculation; 3) ductal obstruction; or, rarely, 4) hormonal deficiencies. Abnormal sperm motility can be due to many factors, such as the presence of a varicocele, anti-sperm antibodies, infections, toxins, and even non-viable sperm. Morphology is the most subjective parameter measured in the semen analysis, but significant variations in morphology often reflect underlying testicular dysfunction. Sometimes no obvious source for abnormally low sperm counts will be found on initial evaluation. This condition has been termed "idiopathic oligospermia." However, a more in-depth search may reveal a source of the problem.

There are several other studies which may aid in the evaluation of infertile male patients. Scrotal ultrasound has been used to measure the size of the testicles, evaluate epididymal or testicular masses, or to confirm the resolution of varicoceles post-operatively. Transrectal ultrasound can be used to search for abnormalities of the seminal vesicles or ejaculatory ducts in patients with azoospermia or low semen volumes. Ultrasound of the kidneys is recommended in patients found to have absent vas deferens, since approximately 20 percent of patients with abnormalities or absence of the seminal vesicles or vas deferens are missing the ipsilateral kidney.

Even though sperm may look normal on semen analysis, they may not function normally. There are many tests that attempt to evaluate sperm function, and these may be valuable in the work-up of select patients.

Anti-sperm antibodies (antibodies to proteins on the surfaces of sperm) are found in 10 to 15 percent of infertile men. These antibodies, which can bind to sperm, have been implicated in impaired semen analyses and are believed to exert an adverse effect on pregnancy. Various tests for anti-sperm antibodies exist.

The treatment of male infertility can be medical or surgical depending on the underlying cause. Specific medical therapy tends to be more successful in patients with hormonal problems. For example, patients with hypothyroidism may have impaired fertility that resolves with replacement of thyroid hormone. Patients with infertility due to testosterone deficiency, or lack of other male hormones, may benefit from testosterone replacement. Elevated levels of the hormone prolactin can also contribute to male factor infertility. The causes of hyperprolactinemia include pituitary tumors, hypothyroidism, and various drugs. Therefore, the treatment of elevated prolactin levels can also involve either medical or surgical therapy. The presence of anti-sperm antibodies in the semen of infertile men has been treated with steroids or some form of sperm processing for use in either intrauterine injection or *in vitro* fertilization (IVF). The treatment of retrograde ejaculation was discussed in Chapter 8; however, as stated previously, specific medical therapy to help close the bladder neck during ejaculation may correct retrograde ejaculation in up to 40 percent of patients.

Occasionally, an infectious cause of infertility may be suspected by the presence of white blood cells on semen analysis. In this case, although infection is usually difficult to document with cultures, many clinicians feel that a trial of antibiotic therapy is warranted. However, there are no controlled studies that demonstrate improved pregnancy rates following antibiotic therapy for idiopathic infertility.

Several different drugs have been used to treat idiopathic oligospermia (low sperm count of unknown origin). This therapy is indicated if the male partner in an infertile marriage has poor semen quality, no known reversible cause, normal hormonal studies, and if his partner has been completely evaluated and optimally treated. Tamoxifen, an anti-estrogen, is believed to result in increased levels of testosterone and, hopefully, improved sperm counts. A dose of 20 mg/day is usually given for up to three to six months. It is usually well tolerated, and pregnancy rates have been reported to range from 11 to 40 percent. Clomiphene citrate is also an anti-estrogen with success rates similar to tamoxifen; however, it has been noted to have more side effects than tamoxifen. Various other drugs have been used in an attempt to improve sperm counts or motility, but their actual benefit remains unclear.

Surgical management of male infertility can be either diagnostic or therapeutic. As stated earlier, testicular biopsy may be indicated to rule out testicular dysfunction; however, a testicular biopsy may also be used to obtain sperm for IVF.

In patients found to have obstruction of the epididymis or vas deferens, various surgical options exist depending on the type and location of the blockage. The incidence of ductal obstruction among infertile men is approximately 7 percent. The causes of ductal obstruction include congenital absence of the ductal system, ductal scarring following infection, vasectomy, and functional obstruction from motility problems in the tubes themselves.

Advances in surgical techniques, as well as IVF, have provided effective treatment options for men born without the vas deferens. Microsurgical epididymal sperm aspiration (MESA) is a technique in which sperm is harvested from the epididymis using a needle or micropipette. Sperm obtained in this fashion can then be utilized for *in vitro* fertilization. This technique has been used primarily for patients born with absence of the vasa deferentia and less frequently for patients with failed reconstructive procedures.

Strictures or obstructions of the vas deferens due to infection or prior surgical trauma can be treated with excision of the obstructed area and reconnection of the patent sections (i.e., vasovasostomy). Epididymal obstructions may require an epididymovasostomy (surgical connection of the epididymis to the patent segment of the vas deferens) or MESA.

Obstruction of the ejaculatory ducts as they pass through the prostate may be congenital or due to prior infections or surgery. This problem can be treated with transurethral resection. In this procedure, the patient is placed under anesthesia and a fiberoptic instrument known as a cystoscope is passed up through the patient's urethra to the area of obstruction at the level of the prostate. The obstructing tissue is then either incised or resected. Improved sperm counts and pregnancy rates have been reported using this technique in patients with ejaculatory duct obstruction. In these cases, the bladder neck needs to be preserved to prevent retrograde ejaculation.

Artificial insemination is a process in which sperm, which has been collected from either the husband (AIH) or an unknown donor (AID), is processed and then injected into the female's uterus at the optimal time in an attempt to achieve a pregnancy. The development of artificial insemination has been linked to advances in semen processing and storage. In addition to artificial insemination, IVF can be used in couples with either associated or solitary male infertility. Pregnancy rates in this population have been reported to be between 20 and 40 percent. As stated prior, up to 30 percent of male patients with azoospermia and significantly elevated levels of follicle stimulating hormone (FSH) can be found to have mature sperm on testis biopsy. Sperm obtained in this fashion could be used for IVF. This procedure offers these couples an alternative to adoption.

Advances in the diagnosis and treatment of male infertility are being made each day. Types of male factor infertility once believed to be untreatable are being managed today with fairly good pregnancy rates. The bottom line is that in this day and age, if you have sperm on a semen analysis, you can probably achieve a pregnancy, depending on how far you are willing to go. Even if no sperm is present on semen analysis, there is a chance sperm may be found in a testis biopsy and, if so, this sperm could be used in IVF to try to achieve a pregnancy. Once the bullet is fired and pregnancy achieved, then the real hard part begins: taking care of the kids. Good luck!

References

1. Gilbert BR, Cooper GW, Goldstein M: "Semen Analysis in the Evaluation of Male Factor Subfertility." *AUA Update Series* 1992; vol. 11, lesson 32.
2. Gilbert BR, Schlegel PN, Goldstein M: "Office Evaluation of the Subfertile Male." *AUA Update Series* 1994; vol. 13, lesson 9.
3. Gilbert BR, Witkin SS, and Goldstein M: "Immunology of Male Infertility." *AUA Update Series* 1990; vol. 9, lesson 8.
4. Gillenwater JY, Grayhack JT, Howards SS, Duckett JW (eds): *Adult and Pediatric Urology*, 3rd ed. St. Louis: Mosby, 1996.
5. Greenberg SH, Lipshultz LI, and Wein AJ: "Experience with 425 Subfertile Male Patients." *J Urol* 1978; 119(4):507-510.
6. Irianni F and Acosta AA: "Evaluation of Male Factor for Assisted Reproduction." *AUA Update Series* 1995; vol. 14, lesson 18.
7. Kim ED, Gilbaugh JH, Patel VR, Turek PJ, and Lipshultz LI: "Testis Biopsies Frequently Demonstrate Sperm in Men with Azoospermia and

Significantly Elevated Follicle Stimulating Hormone Levels." *J Urol* 1997; 157(1):144-146.

8. Van Arsdalen KN and Wessells H: "Surgery of Male Infertility Part II: Procedures for Ductal Obstruction." *AUA Update Series* 1994; vol. 13, lesson 11.

9. Wessells H and Van Arsdalen KN: "Surgery of Male Infertility Part I: Varicocelectomy, Testis Biopsy, and Vasography." *AUA Update Series* 1994; vol. 13, lesson 10.

CHAPTER 12

VASECTOMY

Picture this TV commercial which borrows from another successful ad campaign: A playroom full of toys. Screaming children running all over the room and causing all types of destruction. The camera slowly pulls back and we see that we're looking through a large window. We then see the father, an agonizing look on his face, pressed up against this window as if pleading for help. The screen goes black except for the words: Got Kids? The screen then changes to show the words: Vasectomy! Call 1-800-FOR-A-CUT.

In the United States, approximately 7 percent of all married couples choose vasectomy as their form of birth control, resulting in about 500,000 vasectomies being performed each year. As described in Chapter 4, during the sexual act, sperm travel from the epididymis through the vas deferens (one on each side), become part of the seminal fluid, and are ejaculated through the penis. The purpose of a vasectomy is to obliterate the lumen of each vas deferens (plural is *vasa deferentia*) to prevent the sperm from becoming part of the ejaculate (see Figure 12.1).

Most patients who desire vasectomy have had one or more children and, because they feel that their family is complete, do not want any more. They have usually tried other forms of birth control but want something more permanent. At the time of initial counseling, I usually emphasize that, although vasectomy reversal is possible, it is not 100 percent effective in restoring fertility. Therefore, vasectomy should be considered a permanent form of sterilization. Of note, sperm banking is an option before vasectomy, just in case the patient changes his mind about having more children after the vasectomy.

Vasectomy can be performed in the operating room or in the office. Most patients choose to have it done in the office to keep costs down. Of

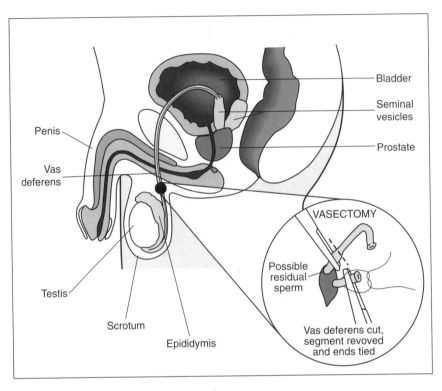

Figure 12-1: The male reproductive system and vasectomy.

course, urologists will differ slightly in how they perform a vasectomy, but following is a general description of the traditional technique.

The patient may be given a prescription for 10 mg. of Valium with instructions to bring the pill to the office on the day of surgery. Some physicians may use an injectable form of a drug similar to Valium to help relax or mildly sedate the patient.

On the morning of the surgery, the patient shaves the hair off his scrotum and a little from the area above his penis. He comes to the office with someone to drive him home. He is instructed to take the Valium 15 to 30 minutes before the procedure. The patient is then placed on the surgery table with his legs up (i.e., like a woman having a baby). The doctor then injects anesthetic on both sides of the penis to numb the testicle and the spermatic cord on each side. These injections feel like bad bee stings. Some researchers have suggested that this blind infiltration of the cord, known as a cord block, may risk damage to the testicle; however, this risk is small, and the benefit of cord block during vasectomy is immense. Personally, I've performed vasectomies both with and without cord block, and most patients tolerate vasectomy better with the cord block.

The nurse then cleans the patient with an antibacterial soap solution and drapes him for surgery. A local anesthetic is injected to numb the skin on each side of the scrotum, and after that, most patients do not feel much more than mild pulling and tugging on the cord. The vas deferens is palpated and fixed to the skin with a special clamp. This can be done in the midline of the scrotum so that only one incision needs to be made, but I like to use one incision on each side of the scrotum to avoid grabbing the same vas deferens twice. It's a personal preference.

A 0.5 cm. to 1.0 cm. incision is made in the skin over the vas deferens. The incision is continued down to the vas, which can be identified by its pearly white appearance. The vas deferens is then separated from the surrounding structures, and a short segment (about 1 inch long) is removed. The lumen of both cut ends of the vas are then cauterized for at least 1 cm. in length. Both ends are also then tied off with a suture. I prefer to separate the two ends into different tissue planes to decrease the risk of their rejoining, an occurrence called recanalization. The incision is closed with absorbable suture, which usually takes a few weeks to dissolve completely. Then the same procedure is performed on the other side.

Some surgeons have tried to avoid ligating (i.e., tying off) the testicular end of the vas by using only intraluminal fulguration. The latter technique involves using electrical current to promote the occlusion, or closure, of the vas. It is believed that this method decreases the risk of chronic pain. However, since some studies have suggested a higher rate of recanalization and vasectomy failure with this method, I usually cut, burn, tie, and separate the two ends into different tissue planes. After all, vasectomy should be considered a reliable permanent procedure, and I want to try to assure that it will be.

The operation usually takes about 20 to 30 minutes, after which the patient is given an instruction sheet for postoperative care. It is recommended to keep the area dry for two days. An ice pack on the wound for 24 hours helps keep swelling to a minimum. No strenuous activity is allowed for one week.

It is recommended that the patient abstain from sexual intercourse for one to two weeks to allow ample time for healing. After these two weeks, the patient can have as much intercourse as he desires. However, until a follow-up semen analysis demonstrates no sperm, protection must be used. This is because sperm can be stored in the seminal vesicles for a while. Patients cannot be cleared for unprotected intercourse until a post-vasectomy semen analysis shows there is no longer sperm. Approximately 80 to 90 percent of males who undergo a vasectomy will be azoospermic after 12 to 15 ejaculations, but even after 20 times a fair amount of patients show some non-motile sperm detected on the follow-up semen analysis. Non-motile sperm seen after a vasectomy usually mean that the patient did not have enough ejaculations to empty his seminal vesicles of sperm. After I started recommending 40 ejaculations before the follow-up semen analysis, achieving azoospermia has not been a problem, and the only complaints have come from the patient's wives.

ALTERNATIVE METHODS OF STERILIZATION

The search for faster, less invasive means of male sterilization began in China. One technique is known as the no-scalpel vasectomy. In this method, a specialized clamp is used to stabilize and fix the vas deferens to the skin. Then, a sharpened, curved clamp is used to puncture the scrotal skin in the midline and deliver the vas deferens out of this wound. The rest of the procedure (i.e., cutting, fulgurating, and/or ligating the vas deferens) is as described for the traditional method. Since the entry site usually contracts down to 2 to 3 mm. by the end of the procedure, no sutures are necessary to close the wound. The no-scalpel technique has two advantages over the traditional method: the risks of bleeding and of local complications are lower, and the patient has less postoperative pain and swelling. The failure rate for this method is similar to that for the traditional one. This technique does require additional training to develop expertise in using the specialized instruments. The no-scalpel technique is now widely used in the United States as well.

In China, studies are being carried out to evaluate the injection of a solution of polyurethane that forms a plug that occludes the lumen of the vas. The vas deferens is fixed to the skin in the usual manner, then a needle is passed into the lumen. Dye is used to assure accurate placement of the needle within the vas lumen. Then, a small volume of the chemical is injected to occlude the lumen of the vas deferens. Aside from the extensive testing and approval of the FDA required to inject chemicals into the human body, the failure rate of this method is presently 2 percent which is unacceptably high. More work needs to be done with this technique.

There are several risks, or possible complications, of vasectomy. They include:

1. Infection: A little redness and swelling is expected, but pain, fever, or purulent discharge is not. Infection occurs in 0.2 to 3 percent of cases and usually resolves with antibiotics.

2. Bleeding: Some bloody drainage and ecchymosis (i.e., black and blue discoloration of the skin) usually occurs. However, if the scrotum swells up like a baseball or softball, the physician needs to be notified because a blood vessel may have opened up. This risk of bleeding is 1 to 2 percent, and approximately 1 in 1000 patients will need to be hospitalized and occasionally will need to have the blood drained surgically.

3. Pain: Once the anesthetic wears off, the patient feels as if he has been kicked in the testicles. He is usually prescribed pain medication, such as Tylenol with codeine. Most patients feel better by the end of the first week, although some take more time and some take less time. Rarely, scrotal or testicular pain persists or recurs intermittently after inter-course. This could be due to involvement of nerves in scar tissue. Usually, this intermittent, chronic pain is the result of the vas deferens reacting to the obstruction of its lumen. This condition which can also be associated with fullness and pain in the epididymis is called *conges-tive epididymitis*, and it is usually treated with anti-inflammatory medi-cation, such as ibuprofen, warm sitz baths, and scrotal support until the pain resolves. Approximately 1 out of every 10,000 patients will

experience chronic testicular pain significant enough to require inter-vention, such as vasectomy reversal.

4. Spermatic granuloma: Occasionally, sperm from the vas deferens leak out during or after the vasectomy. The body can react to this sperm and create a hard knot of inflammatory tissue that can be painful and might need to be removed.

5. Loss of testicles: Any time an operation involves the spermatic cord, the blood supply to the testicle can be compromised, and the testicle could infarct and subsequently shrivel up into a little nubbin of tissue. For that to happen on one side is rare. For it to happen on both sides in the same patient is extremely rare.

6. Failure of the procedure: Vasectomy failure occurs 0.1 to 0.3 percent of the time. This can occur from recanalization or, rarely, from the presence of two vasa deferentia on one side which was not noticed at the time of initial examination or at vasectomy. The presence of motile sperm on the post-vasectomy semen analysis heralds failure. If azoospermia (no sperm) fails to occur within three months after the vasectomy, the procedure should be repeated. Although recanalization has been reported up to 17 years after vasectomy, the vast majority occur within the first 6 weeks.

7. Questionable association of vasectomy with prostate cancer: Recently, data suggesting an increased association between vasectomy and pros-tate cancer have been presented. The assessment of evidence supporting this association and other more recent studies indicate that any causal relationship between vasectomy and the risk of prostate cancer is unlikely.

Long-term studies of vasectomized males, who have been followed for up to 25 years in cohorts of up to 10,000 males and in control groups, demonstrate no evidence for a significant increase in any systemic disorder after vasectomy.

A few myths and common misconceptions regarding vasectomy need to be addressed. First of all, although vasectomy will hopefully make one sterile, it will not have any effect on potency. That is, a male's ability to get erections will not be affected by vasectomy. Also, there will be no noticeable decrease in the amount of fluid ejaculated, since most of the seminal fluid which the male ejaculates during intercourse is produced by the seminal vesicles and the prostate gland.

In summary, vasectomy is a simple and effective method of permanent contraception. It is usually well tolerated, and the overwhelming evidence to date indicates that vasectomy is safe and not associated with any serious, long-term adverse effects. The bottom line is —if you want to avoid a visit from the stork above, get the cut below.

References

1. Gillenwater JY, Grayhack JT, Howards SS, Duckett JW (eds.): *Adult and Pediatric Urology*, 3rd ed. St. Louis: Mosby, 1996.
2. Schlegel PN and Goldstein M: "Vasectomy." *AUA Update Series* 1992; vol. 11, lesson 13.

CHAPTER 13

VASECTOMY REVERSAL

Approximately 500,000 American males have vasectomies each year. It is estimated that up to 6 percent of these men will seek reversal (vasovasostomy), the most common reason being divorce and subsequent remarriage. Other reasons for vasectomy reversal include death of a child or, rarely, for relief of the post-vasectomy pain syndrome. As discussed in the earlier chapter on infertility, vasovasostomy may also be performed to treat infertility caused by ductal obstruction. In this chapter, the techniques, possible complications, and success rates of vasovasostomy will be discussed.

There are many methods for performing a vasovasostomy, and no one way has been proven to be superior. Surgeon experience is crucial. The surgery itself can be performed under local, spinal, or general anesthesia. The use of microscopic magnification has improved the results of vasovasostomy. Some surgeons use optical loupes (a form of magnifying eyeglasses), instead of employing the operative microscope.

After the patient is cleaned and sterile drapes have been placed for surgery, vertical incisions are made in the anterolateral aspects of the scrotum (one side at a time). Dissection is continued until both ends of the vas deferens are mobilized. The scarred areas of each end of the vas are sharply cut until a normal lumen is seen on both sides. Fluid from the testicular end of the vas is aspirated and examined under a microscope. The prognosis is better if spermatozoa are present.

The two ends of the vas are approximated and sutured together. Some surgeons suture the vas together with predominately one layer of suture, while other surgeons prefer a two-layer anastomosis. There is no convincing evidence that either method yields better results. The same procedure is then performed on the other side.

Some new techniques that have been applied to vasovasostomy in attempts to decrease operating time and prevent sperm leakage include: laser assistance to "weld" the vas ends together after the one-layer closure; and fibrin glue vasal anastomosis after suture closure to try to seal the outer layer of the vas closure. Patency rates (i.e., the chance that the lumen between the two ends of the vas deferens will stay open after being sutured together) are not significantly different from the standard anastomoses, and the significance of sperm leakage is not known since sperm granuloma experimentally do not appear to adversely affect patency or fertility. These newer techniques need more study to determine their role in vasovasostomy.

The procedure is done on a day-surgery basis, so patients usually go home the day of surgery. Patients are advised to use an ice pack for 24 hours to help keep swelling to a minimum, and a scrotal support is suggested until discomfort with walking subsides. Tylenol, or Tylenol with codeine, is usually sufficient for pain relief. Patients are able to return to work within a few days, but they are advised to avoid heavy lifting and ejaculation for two weeks.

Some risks of vasovasostomy include: 1) infection; 2) bleeding; 3) pain (which usually resolves by the end of the first week); 4) sperm granuloma (see Chapter 12); and 5) failure to restore patency of the vas deferens as evidenced by azoospermia on the post-operative semen analysis. This last situation can occur due to obstruction at the level of the epididymis. After vasectomy, sperm is still produced by the testicles. Pressure from sperm accumulation can cause "blow-outs," or ruptures, of the epididymal tubules which may result in inflammation and scarring of these tubules. Over time, the epididymis can become blocked with scar tissue from these episodes, and in these instances, even after vasectomy reversal, patency is not possible unless an epididymovasostomy (surgical procedure in which the vas deferens is attached to the epididymis) is performed. This situation can be seen in approximately 2 percent of initial vasovasostomies.

Another risk of vasovasostomy is delayed obstruction of the vas deferens with progressive scarring after patency is initially confirmed by semen analysis. The risk of this complication has been reported to be about 12 percent. In an attempt to correct this problem, either a repeat vasovasostomy or an epididymovasostomy would need to be performed. Further risks include the failure to achieve a pregnancy despite documentation of patency; and heart attack, stroke, or death, which are risks of anesthesia but rarely occur in young, healthy men.

Patency rates after vasovasostomy have been reported to be approximately 98 percent, but may be lower in patients undergoing repeat vasectomy reversal. Pregnancy rates after vasovasostomy have been reported to be as high as 60 percent. However, the time between vasectomy and vasectomy reversal appears to affect success rates. The best results have been seen in patients who underwent vasovasostomy less than six years after vasectomy. If the procedure is performed more than ten years after vasectomy, reported pregnancy rates drop to between 10 and 30 percent.

Although vasectomy should be considered a permanent procedure by those choosing it as their method of birth control, life has a way of making people change their minds. Vasovasostomy is a well-tolerated, relatively low-risk operation with fairly good success rates for those very brave people who decide to have more children after vasectomy.

References

1. Gilbert BR, Witkin SS, and Goldstein M: "Immunology of Male Infertility." *AUA Update Series* 1990; vol. 9, lesson 8.
2. Gillenwater JY, Grayhack JT, Howards SS, Duckett JW (eds.): *Adult and Pediatric Urology*, 3rd ed. St. Louis: Mosby, 1996.
3. Matthews GJ, McGee KE, and Goldstein M: "Microsurgical Reconstruction Following Failed Vasectomy Reversal." *J Urol* 1997; 157(3):844-846.
4. Myers SA, Mershon CE, and Fuchs EF: "Vasectomy Reversal For Treatment of the Post-Vasectomy Pain Syndrome." *J Urol* 1997; 157(2):518-520.
5. Van Arsdalen KN and Wessells H: "Surgery of Male Infertility Part II: Procedures for Ductal Obstruction." *AUA Update Series* 1994; vol. 13, lesson 11.

CHAPTER 14

SEXUALLY
TRANSMITTED DISEASES

*"Intercourse is the most dangerous sexual act.
One huge risk is pregnancy itself. Of course,
Mother Nature would have a tough time with that
one. She did not foresee a time when reproducing
the species would be the least of our problems; we
already have more people than we know what to do
with. Conception is the goal only a tiny proportion
of times men and women get together sexually.
Disease is another problem. Although it's true that
most sexually transmitted diseases can be
transmitted orally, the main risk is intercourse."*

Modified from B. Zilbergeld,
The New Male Sexuality,
Bantam Books, 1992.

With the freedom of the sexual revolution came an increase in the prevalence and types of sexually transmitted diseases (STDs). Aside from the well-known venereal diseases, such as syphilis and gonorrhea, there has been an increase in the incidence and prevalence of urethritis, genital herpes, and acquired immunodeficiency syndrome (AIDS). The increase in STDs is an important health problem due to the consequences of these diseases: spontaneous abortion, ectopic pregnancy, pelvic inflammatory disease (PID), infertility, cervical carcinoma, and death. It is estimated that up to 50 percent of the U.S. population will acquire an STD by age 35. Of note, 60 percent of patients with one sexually transmitted disease can be found to have another. In order to avoid a ping-pong effect (i.e., passing the disease back and forth), it is recommended that all sexual partners of patients with an STD be evaluated and treated. This chapter will review some of the more common STDs.

URETHRITIS

Urethritis —literally, inflammation of the urethra— represents the response of the urethra to irritation of any cause. Such inflammation results in the classic symptoms of urethral discharge, usually accompanied by burning on urination or an itchy sensation in the penis. Urethritis has been around for as long as men and women have been "getting around."

There are numerous causes of urethritis, many of which are non-sexually transmitted; however, this section will deal only with the sexually transmitted causes of urethritis.

Nongonococcal Urethritis

Nongonococcal urethritis (NGU) is believed to be the most common type of urethritis. The organism *Chlamydia trachomatis* is believed to be the most common cause of NGU in men. It has a prolonged incubation period of 5 to 21 days and usually produces a watery or mucoid, whitish discharge, with or without dysuria (burning on urination). The real health problem is that 50 percent of chlamydial infections are asymptomatic, so these patients transmit the infection without even knowing it.

The diagnosis of NGU requires the exclusion of gonorrhea and demonstration of a true inflammation of the urethra by microscopic examination of the urethral discharge. It is difficult to culture chlamydia, but attempts are sometimes made. Various antibiotics are used to treat NGU. Tetracycline or doxycycline are usually given for seven days. Treatment failure can be expected in up to 40 percent of men due to trichomonas urethritis (another STD caused by the organism *Trichomonas vaginalis*) which usually resolves with a course of metronidazole (Flagyl).

Gonococcal Urethritis (Gonorrhea)

The word "gonorrhea" was termed by the Greek physician and writer Galen, around 130-201 A.D., and is a combination of the word *gonus* (seed) and *rhoea* (flow). Gonorrhea literally means "leakage of semen." Eventually it was recognized that the discharge was pus, not semen, and that urethritis followed intercourse with an infected woman. This led to efforts to control venereal diseases by regulating prostitution. In fact, during the

Middle Ages, prostitutes in Paris were restricted to domiciles called "clapiers" (hence, the origin of the term "clap").

Gonorrhea is one of the most common communicable diseases. It is estimated that as many as 2.5 million infections occur in the United States each year. The incubation period for gonorrhea is two to five days in the majority of cases, and most often it produces a purulent, yellowish, urethral discharge with dysuria. Twenty-five percent of infected males have a nonpurulent, mucoid discharge as in NGU, and 20 percent can be asymptomatic. Complications of gonorrhea in the male include epididymitis, prostatitis, and urethral strictures.

The diagnosis of gonorrhea is based on a history of sexual contact, a purulent urethral discharge, demonstration of the organism on microscopic examination and/or culture of a specimen obtained from the patient's urethra.

Penicillin was a time-honored treatment that is no longer recommended due to the increasing resistance of the gonococcus to this antibiotic. Single-dose treatments of various antibiotics (e.g., ceftriaxone, ofloxacin, or ciprofloxacin) are usually given; however, since up to 45 percent of men with gonorrhea will also be infected with *Chlamydia trachomatis*, it is recommended that patients with gonorrhea also be treated for NGU. Therefore, in addition to the treatment for gonorrhea described above, a seven day course of tetracycline or doxycycline is now added. Follow-up evaluation one week after treatment is recommended for all patients in order to diagnose and treat any persistent infections that may be due to resistant organisms or poor patient compliance.

SYPHILIS

Syphilis, caused by the organism *Treponema pallidum*, has been called "the great imitator" because of its varied manifestations as it progresses through different stages. The organism usually gains entrance through the intact skin of the penis in the male. Primary syphilis is characterized by the chancre, a painless penile ulcer with indurated borders and a clear discharge which appears 10 to 30 days following infection. It is usually solitary and lasts for one to five weeks. The secondary stage appears two to ten weeks later as a generalized rash involving the palms and soles, the oral cavity, and the anogenital areas. Enlargement of lymph nodes frequently accompanies the rash. These lesions also heal spontaneously. Latent syphilis, or the third stage, is without signs or symptoms until it is untreatable. The organism spreads to all organs, especially the cardiovascular and central nervous systems. The patient remains potentially infectious for approximately the first two years of this stage.

The diagnosis of syphilis is made by identifying the organism by microscopic examination of fluid from a chancre. There are also various blood tests which can be used to confirm the diagnosis (e.g., RPR, VDRL, or certain antibody tests).

Penicillin has been, and remains, the drug of choice for syphilis. Tetracycline or erythromycin are alternatives for penicillin-allergic patients.

GENITAL HERPES SIMPLEX

The term herpes originated from the Greek verb meaning "to creep." To date, seven human herpes viruses have been identified. Infection with herpes simplex virus-type I (HSV-1) and herpes simplex virus-type II (HSV-2) may cause genital or oral lesions. It is estimated that between 270,000 and 600,000 new cases of genital herpes occur each year in the United States. HSV infection occurs by close contact with a person who is shedding virus particles. The virus travels up sensory nerve roots and can remain dormant for long periods of time. Viral shedding occurs primarily from ruptured vesicular skin lesions but can also occur during asymptomatic periods.

Initial infection with HSV is often associated with fever, headache, malaise, or enlarged lymph nodes. Recurrent infections are generally less severe and are manifested primarily by the characteristic skin lesions: grouped vesicles, erosions, or crusted ulcers which are painful and usually last 4 to 15 days. The average number of recurrences is about four per year. The diagnosis of herpes is confirmed by culture of the virus particles from fluid obtained from a skin lesion.

The key to the treatment of herpes at the present time is control of symptomatic episodes. Oral acyclovir (trade name Zovirax) is not virucidal or curative, but it does block viral replication and is clinically effective in treating primary and recurrent infections by decreasing their severity, frequency, and duration. Acyclovir can be administered intravenously in severe infections. Some newer drugs used to treat HSV include: valacyclovir (trade name Valtrex) and famciclovir (Famvir). These drugs are related to acyclovir, so they have similar side effects, the most common being headache and nausea. They are taken orally; however, since they require less frequent dosing than acyclovir, they are more convenient for the patient. Currently, the development of an HSV vaccine is an area of intense research.

There are several other diseases which can cause lesions in the genital area, including chancroid, lymphogranuloma venereum, granuloma inguinale, and scabies. These need to be distinguished to be treated appropriately. Basically, any persistent lesion in the genital area is not normal and usually requires medical evaluation and treatment.

ACQUIRED IMMUNODEFICIENCY SYNDROME

Currently, it is estimated by the Center for Disease Control (CDC) that one in every 250 persons in the United States is infected with the human immunodeficiency virus (HIV), the causative organism for acquired immunodeficiency syndrome, or AIDS. This disease has now become the leading cause of death among adults from 25 to 44 years of age.

The virus is spread by sexual contact with an infected individual, by sharing a contaminated needle, by receipt of infected blood or blood products, and from mother to unborn child. Anal intercourse, particularly for the receptive partner, carries the most risk for sexual transmission of HIV. The largest number of individuals with AIDS remains men who have sex with men; however, recent trends indicate that the AIDS epidemic is increasing among injecting drug users and persons infected through heterosexual contact. This increase in heterosexual transmission is resulting in more cases being reported among women.

After a person has been infected with HIV, the peripheral blood contains large numbers of infected lymphocytes (which are a particular type of infection-fighting, white blood cell). During this period, usually between two weeks and three months, there is widespread dissemination of HIV throughout the body. At this time, blood tests for HIV screening may be negative. But by the end of six months, more than 95 percent of all infected individuals will have positive blood tests indicated by the presence of HIV antibodies.

HIV can produce a spectrum of clinical manifestations ranging from asymptomatic to severe immunodeficiency and neurologic disease. There are four general categories of disease manifestation: 1) opportunistic infections (e.g., *pneumocystis carinii* pneumonia); 2) cancers (e.g., lymphoma, Kaposi's sarcoma); 3) neurologic disease (e.g., AIDS neuropathy); and 4) autoimmune phenomena (e.g., blood abnormalities, especially decreased white blood cell counts).

The diagnosis of AIDS is suspected by a past history of "risky" behavior and the finding of manifestations of the disease on evaluation. It is confirmed by various blood tests that search for antibodies to the virus.

The number of antiviral agents used to treat HIV infection has increased dramatically in the past few years. Unfortunately, although significant amounts of time and money are being invested in the area of AIDS research, a cure for this disease has yet to be found. To date, the diagnosis of AIDS carries a grave prognosis. Therefore, at the present time, the treatment for AIDS is preventative. HIV transmission can be prevented by eliminating or revising behaviors that put individuals at risk for infection. Aside from sexual abstinence, reducing the number of sexual partners and using latex condoms during anal, oral, or vaginal intercourse can significantly reduce the risk of HIV transmission. The additional use of spermicides may reduce transmission even further. Individuals should not share needles. The CDC also advises against the sharing of personal items, such as toothbrushes, razors, or sexual devices that may be contaminated with blood, semen, or vaginal fluids.

CONDYLOMA ACUMINATA: WARTS

Genital warts, also known as venereal warts, fig warts (because of their resemblance to figs), or condyloma acuminata, are cauliflower-like lesions of the skin caused by human papillomavirus (HPV). These viruses also cause warts in other locations, including palms and soles, voice box, and in oral and anal areas. It is estimated that approximately 30 million people in the United States are infected with genital HPV, and that approximately 300,000 initial medical visits each year are due to HPV infection. Recently, public concern over genital warts has increased due to the association of HPV infection with various malignancies, especially cervical cancer.

Epidemiological evidence supports the idea that genital warts are transmitted sexually in the majority of cases. After infection, which most probably begins with trauma to the skin allowing the virus to reach and infect cells, there is rapid duplication of the virus. Released viral particles are then transmitted by autoinoculation to other anatomic areas and to other persons who contact the infected site. Approximately two-thirds of sexual contacts of infected patients develop similar lesions. The incubation period of the virus is usually four to six weeks, but may be as long as nine months in some cases.

To date, more than 75 distinct HPV types have been described. These are referred to as genotypes. Over 20 HPV genotypes infect the urogenital tract. Aside from causing genital condyloma, HPV is important due to its association with certain genital cancers including cervical cancer, urethral cancer, anal cancer, and penile cancer. "Classic" genital warts are usually caused by HPV types 6 and 11 which carry a low risk for malignancy. HPV 16 and 18 are associated with a high risk for malignancy.

Warts tend to occur in areas where the skin is thin, or on mucous membranes. Approximately 5 percent of patients will develop urethral disease, 90 percent of which will involve only the external meatus and distal penile urethra. These patients usually have a history of prior non-urethral involvement. Symptoms of intraurethral warts can include urethral discharge, dysuria, splaying of the urine stream, blood-spotting on undergarments, or blood at the beginning of urination (initial hematuria).

The diagnosis of genital warts is usually straightforward. Patients typically complain of a cauliflower-like lesion on their penis or scrotum. Lesions may also be soft, fleshy, and vascular. A search is made of the entire anogenital area. Acetic-acid mixtures (the "vinegar test") have been used to help locate infected cells when the classic lesions are not yet apparent to the naked eye (subclinical infection). After a few minutes of exposure to the mixture, the infected areas develop a whitish discoloration. However, this staining test is nonspecific, and the significance of subclinical infection is controversial. HPV does not grow in cell culture, and the only reliable way to accurately detect and determine the type of HPV infection is with sophisticated tests involving DNA analysis.

The treatment of genital warts frequently depends on the size and the number of lesions, but the options include topical agents, immunotherapy, cryotherapy, electrofulguration, laser ablation, and surgical excision. Caustic agents, such as 10 to 20 percent podophyllin in compound tincture of benzoin or podofilox, are traditional agents, but skin irritation and pain are common adverse side effects and recurrence rates are high with only a 30 percent cure rate. The topical agent 5-fluorouracil has been used for intraurethral warts as well, as have interferons, which are naturally occurring proteins with antiviral activity. Interferon has been injected systemically and/or intralesionally in attempts to eradicate warts by boosting the host's immune system. Systemic interferon has been reported to decrease the risk of recurrence when used in conjunction with other treatment modalities. More study is needed to determine the efficacy of intralesional interferon injection.

Freezing of warts with liquid nitrogen, known as cryotherapy, has been shown to have a good success rate, approaching 90 percent cure. Electrofulguration has also been shown to have acceptable results. Surgical excision is especially useful with large lesions. In rare cases, skin grafts may be necessary to cover large surgical defects. Recently, laser fulguration of warts has demonstrated excellent success rates and acceptable cosmetic results. Laser ablation is also useful in the treatment of intraurethral lesions. Recurrence rates after laser therapy have been reported to be as low as 7.5 percent at one to two years follow-up.

Given the increased risk of cervical cancer with HPV infection, it is recommended that female partners of patients with genital warts undergo a genital examination by their physician to rule out HPV infection. It is also recommended that patients with genital condyloma use a condom until their warts are eradicated.

Since the most common complication of the treatment of genital warts is recurrent lesions or reinfection, regular medical follow-up or frequent self-examination after treatment is crucial. The bottom line about genital warts can be found in the words of the famous horror-fiction writer, Stephen King, "Sometimes they come back."

References

1. Gillenwater JY, Grayhack JT, Howards SS, Duckett JW (eds.): *Adult and Pediatric Urology*, 3rd ed. St. Louis: Mosby, 1996.
2. Macfarlane MT: *Urology for the House Officer*, 2nd ed., Baltimore: Williams and Wilkins, 1995.
3. Mellinger BC: "Human Papillomavirus in the Male: An Overview." *AUA Update Series* 1994; vol. 13, lesson 13.
4. Pariser DM, Pariser RJ, and Pariser H: "Sexually Transmitted Diseases 1991: Diagnosis and Treatment for the Practicing Clinician." *AUA Update Series* 1991; vol. 10, lesson 29.
5. Zilbergeld B: *The New Male Sexuality*, New York: Bantam Books, 1992.

CHAPTER 15

EPIDIDYMITIS

One cause of testicular pain has already been discussed in the chapter on torsion (see Chapter 3). This chapter will review one of the more common causes of testicular pain.

As seen in Figure 15-1, the epididymis is that convoluted part of the sperm-carrying tube that is closely applied to the posterior aspect of the

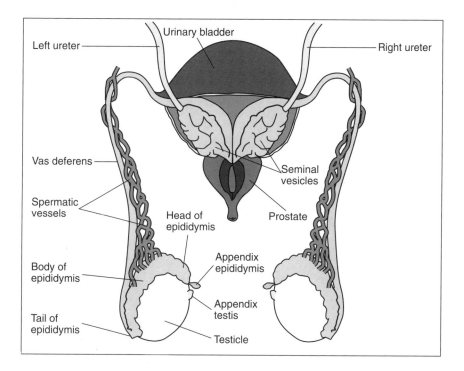

Figure 15-1: *Posterior view of the anatomical relationship of the testis, epididymis, and vas deferens.*

testis. It is composed of the head (upper part), a body (middle part), and a tail end (lower part). It eventually straightens to become the vas deferens which leads to the ejaculatory duct which, in turn, empties into the prostatic portion of the urethra.

Acute epididymitis refers to inflammation, pain, and swelling of the epididymis of less than six weeks duration. Chronic epididymitis involves long-standing pain in the epididymis and testicle, usually without swelling, and can be the result of several episodes of acute epididymitis.

Just as sperm can travel from the epididymis up to the urethra during the sexual act, bacteria can travel from the urethra down to the epididymis. It is believed that the majority of cases of epididymitis are acquired by the retrograde spread of bacteria down the vas deferens from the urethra. In sexually active men under the age of 35, sexually transmitted organisms such as *N. gonorrhea* or *C. trachomatis* are usually responsible for most cases of epididymitis. In children and men older than 35, non-sexually transmitted bacteria are more frequently found to be the cause. Some systemic diseases, such as tuberculosis, can also result in epididymal inflammation. Rarely, a chemical epididymitis may occur secondary to the caustic effect of urine which is forced down the vas into the epididymis. The anti-arrhythmic drug amiodarone has been shown to be selectively concentrated in the epididymis. This can occasionally result in epididymal inflammation which usually resolves with decreasing the dose of amio-darone.

The diagnosis of epididymitis is usually made from the history, physical exam, and a urinalysis consistent with infection. Patients typically present with heaviness and a dull ache in the affected testicle. This pain can radiate up to the ipsilateral flank. Early on, the epididymis can be distinguished from the testicle and is found to be markedly swollen and tender to the touch. Eventually, as the inflammatory process progresses, a warm, red, enlarged scrotal mass develops and the epididymis and testicle become indistinguish-able. Fever and chills may also develop. An examination of the patient's urine will usually reveal bacteria and white blood cells (i.e., pus cells).

The treatment of acute epididymitis involves several measures: 1) antibiotics directed at the specific etiologic organisms; 2) bed rest, or no strenuous activity, and scrotal elevation to help keep pain and swelling to a minimum; 3) pain medication (e.g., Tylenol with codeine); and 4) oral anti-inflammatory medication (e.g., ibuprofen). Complete resolution of pain and swelling may take several weeks to months. The presence of epididymitis in children less than 10 years of age and in older men is uncommon and suggests a possible structural abnormality of the urinary tract. In these cases, a urologic evaluation with x-rays and cystoscopy may be recommended.

Complications from acute epididymitis include: 1) abscess formation, which usually requires removal of the testicle as part of the operation to drain the collection of pus; 2) testicular infarction, which can occur if significant swelling compromises the blood supply to the testicle; 3) infertility, due to obstruction of the epididymis by scarring from the inflammatory process; and 4) chronic epididymitis/chronic pain.

Chronic testicular pain, also known as chronic orchialgia, is defined as intermittent or constant testicular pain, either unilateral or bilateral, which lasts three months or longer and which interferes with the patient's daily activities so as to make him seek medical attention. Patients with this problem typically present with complaints of testicular discomfort with a normal physical examination.

Testicular pain can originate from one of three areas: 1) local (from pathology in the scrotum); 2) inguinal (from abnormalities in the groin that affect the nerves supplying the testes and scrotum (e.g., hernia)); and 3) retroperitoneal (from pathology involving the kidney). Since the nerve supplies of the kidney and testicle arise from the same level of the spinal cord, kidney pain can sometimes be referred to the ipsilateral testicle. Therefore, when patients present with chronic testicular pain, the history, physical examination, and laboratory studies need to take into account these three areas. If no obvious source of the pain is found on initial evaluation, a 14-day trial of antibiotics and anti-inflammatory medications is usually recommended first. The antibiotic is used just in case the patient has a low-grade epididymitis not manifested on urinalysis or culture. The anti-inflammatory drug is recommended to treat any possible low-grade inflammatory process involving the testicle.

For patients who fail to respond to antibiotics and anti-inflammatory agents, a more in-depth search for intrascrotal or renal pathology can be performed with an ultrasound of the scrotum and kidneys. If this evaluation fails to reveal a source of the pain, various methods have been used to relieve the patient's pain or help him deal with it. Some options include: 1) injection of local anesthesia into the spermatic cord on the affected side (i.e., cord block); 2) biofeedback training or psychotherapy which may be available at a pain clinic; 3) microsurgical ablation of the nerve supplying the testicle; and, only as a last resort, 4) orchiectomy (removing the affected testicle). It should be noted that only 50 to 70 percent of patients with chronic testicular pain have relief of that pain after orchiectomy, since some patients can subsequently experience "phantom pain."

Chronic testicular pain can be frustrating to both the patient and the physician; however, with a thorough evaluation and a rational management plan, some relief can usually be achieved. As for acute testicular pain, it is imperative to differentiate epididymitis from torsion promptly, since any delay in the appropriate treatment of torsion can result in loss of the patient's testicle. The bottom line is that testicular pain is not normal and requires immediate medical evaluation and management.

References

1. Davis BE and Noble MJ: "Analysis and Management of Chronic Orchialgia." *AUA Update Series* 1992; vol. 11, lesson 2.
2. Gillenwater JY, Grayhack JT, Howards SS, Duckett JW (eds.): *Adult and Pediatric Urology*, 3rd ed. St. Louis: Mosby, 1996.
3. Macfarlane MT: *Urology for the House Officer*, 2nd ed. Baltimore: Williams and Wilkins, 1995.
4. Schneider R and Williams MA: "Pediatric Urology in the Emergency Department. *AUA Update Series* 1997; vol. 16, lesson 20.

CHAPTER 16

PROSTATITIS

The prostate is an accessory sex gland that sits just below the bladder and through which passes the urethra (see Figure 16-1). Some of its secretions help to liquefy the semen; however, its main claim to fame is the problems it can cause with aging, namely prostate cancer, benign prostatic hyperplasia (BPH), and prostatitis.

The term *prostatitis* is used to describe inflammatory conditions involving the prostate gland, but some patients with unexplained symptoms believed to emanate from the prostate are occasionally labeled with this condition, correctly or incorrectly. Prostatitis has been classified into different syndromes based predominately on the presence or absence of infection or inflammation in the gland (see Table 16-1).

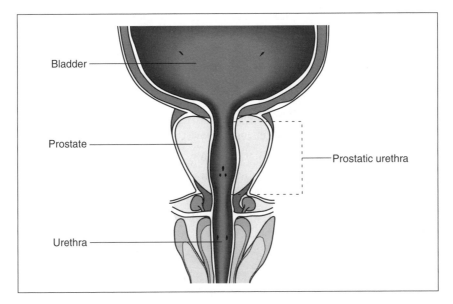

Figure 16-1: *Schematic drawing of the lower urinary tract.*

Table 16-1: Classification of Prostatitis			
Type	Systemic Signs (fever, chills, malaise)	Culture Positive	Evidence of Inflammation	Pain in Prostate
Acute bacterial prostatitis	+	+	+	+
Chronic bacterial prostatitis	-	+	+	+
Nonbacterial prostatitis	-	-	+	+
Pelviperineal pain	-	-	-	+

Acute bacterial prostatitis is believed to be caused by bacteria introduced into the urethra, presumably after vaginal or rectal inoculation during sexual intercourse. It presents with sudden onset of chills, high fever, low back pain, and perineal pain (pain or burning in the area between the scrotum and the anal opening). Patients also usually complain of frequent urination, burning on urination (dysuria), and varying degrees of obstructive voiding symptoms. Some patients may perceive a burning in the anal area as well. Generalized symptoms, such as malaise and joint pain, can also be experienced. The prostate is exquisitely tender and swollen on rectal examination, and bacterial organisms can usually be cultured from the patient's voided urine.

The treatment for acute bacterial prostatitis is a one month course of oral antibiotics. This prolonged antibiotic regimen is recommended in an attempt to prevent chronic infection, known as chronic bacterial prostatitis. In cases of severe infection, patients may need to be hospitalized for intravenous antibiotics until the infection is under control. After this, the patient is sent home on oral antibiotics to complete the full one month treatment course. Occasionally, bacteria in acute bacterial prostatitis can spread down the vas deferens and cause epididymitis. On other occasions, especially if there is a delay in seeking medical attention and the acute bacterial prostatitis is left untreated, a localized collection of pus can develop within the prostate gland. This condition, known as a prostatic abscess, usually requires surgical drainage.

Chronic bacterial prostatitis has a variable presentation; however, it is usually characterized by relatively asymptomatic periods between episodes of recurrent infection. It is one of the most common causes of recurrent urinary tract infections in men. To understand this condition better, one can view the prostate as a sponge with many small spaces. Once bacteria get into the gland and can "hide" in all those spaces, it can be difficult to get rid of all the bacteria. These organisms can then cause recurrent infections. It has also been suggested that impairment of the immune system can predispose patients to chronic bacterial prostatitis.

Most patients with chronic bacterial prostatitis complain of frequency of micturition (urination) and dysuria with genital, perineal, or anal pain. Systemic symptoms, such as fever, chills, or malaise, are unusual. Organisms are usually cultured from the prostatic secretions which also usually show evidence of prostatic inflammation. The treatment of choice for chronic bacterial prostatitis is long-term antibiotic therapy for approximately eight to twelve weeks. This has a cure rate of 60 to 92 percent. The problem is that frequent recurrence is common. It has been suggested that patients who have recurrent episodes may benefit from prolonged courses of suppressive doses of antibiotics to prevent recurrent urinary tract infections. In stubborn cases, an aggressive transurethral resection of the prostate (TURP, the "roto-rooter job") has been attempted with a reported success rate of approximately 30 percent.

Nonbacterial prostatitis is the most common prostatitis syndrome, and although an infectious etiology has been suggested, its cause is unknown. Patients typically present with voiding problems, such as frequency of micturition and dysuria, as well as with genital or perineal pain. The prostatic fluid will usually contain inflammatory cells, but cultures will be negative. In these patients, since there has been some question of an infectious etiology, a trial of antibiotics for two to four weeks is reasonable. If the patient's symptoms persist despite antibiotics, further treatment usually consists of sitz baths, anti-inflammatory agents, such as ibuprofen, or a trial of Valium.

Other treatments that have been used to manage nonbacterial prostatitis with some success include: 1) allopurinol; 2) alpha-blockers, such as Hytrin, Cardura, Flomax, or Minipress, in an attempt to relieve spasms of the muscles in the pelvis and around the prostate; 3) pollen extract, also known as Cernilton; and 4) transurethral microwave thermotherapy (TUMT), which involves heating the prostate gland with microwave energy (see Chapter 20 on benign prostatic hyperplasia (BPH) for more information about TUMT).

Pelviperineal pain, also known as prostatodynia or prostadynia, is used to describe a condition seen in patients, typically 20 to 45 years of age, who complain of abnormal urinary flow, frequency, and pain in the lower back or perineum, but who show no evidence of inflammation in their prostatic fluid and who have negative cultures and no history of documented urinary tract infections. Their symptoms are often associated with stress or long periods of sitting. It has been suggested that problems with muscles and nerves in the area of the bladder outlet and prostatic urethra may be involved in this condition. Therefore, drugs that relax muscles in this area, such as Hytrin, Cardura, Flomax, or Minipress, have been recommended in an attempt to relieve this problem. In addition, pollen extract, hot baths, anti-inflammatory medications, dietary restriction of caffeine, alcohol, and spicy foods, and even biofeedback and other behavior modification techniques have been used successfully to treat some patients with pelviperineal pain. Transurethral microwave thermotherapy (TUMT) has also been used to treat patients with this problem, but it has been suggested that patients with prostatodynia are less likely to respond to TUMT than patients with nonbacterial prostatitis.

Some patients have asked whether taking zinc can protect against the development of prostatitis. A zinc-containing protein called prostatic antibacterial factor (PAF) does appear to be a very important infection-fighting chemical in the prostate, in that the concentration of PAF has been shown to be depressed in the prostatic fluid of men with chronic bacterial prostatitis. However, the concentration of zinc in the prostate is not affected by increasing the oral intake of zinc. Therefore, it is doubtful that oral zinc supplement intake will have a significant beneficial effect on a person's prostate.

The prostatitis syndromes can result in similar symptoms, but can usually be differentiated for appropriate treatment. There are also other prostatic and nonprostatic sources of voiding problems, such as cancer or other inflammatory conditions. It's important to remember that not all that burns is prostatitis; in other words, patients with voiding problems need to be medically evaluated and treated.

References

1. Britton JJ, Jr. and Carson CC: "Prostatitis." *AUA Update Series* 1998; vol. 17, lesson 20.
2. Gillenwater JY, Grayhack JT, Howards SS, Duckett JW (eds.): *Adult and Pediatric Urology*, 3rd ed. St. Louis: Mosby, 1996.
3. Lim DJ and Schaeffer AJ: "Prostatitis Syndromes." *AUA Update Series* 1993; vol. 12, lesson 1.
4. Macfarlane MT: *Urology for the House Officer*, 2nd ed. Baltimore: Williams and Wilkins, 1995.

CHAPTER 17

SCROTAL MASSES

You're taking a shower and feel a lump in your scrotum, or you and your partner are engaged in foreplay, and she feels a scrotal lump that you hadn't noticed before. Thinking you have cancer, you immediately call your doctor. . .

Even though the majority of scrotal masses are benign, discovering a mass in the scrotum makes one anxious! Prompt medical evaluation is needed to rule out life-threatening cancers and any other threats to testicular function. This chapter reviews the anatomy of the scrotum and describes some of the most common causes of scrotal masses.

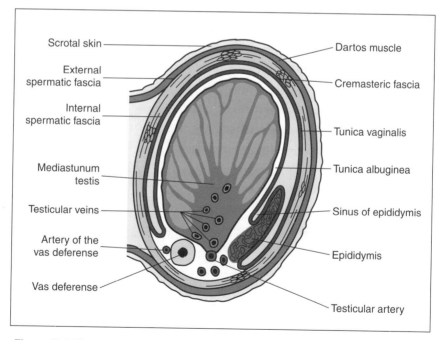

Figure 17-1: *Transverse section of the testis.*

ANATOMY

As seen in Figure 17-1, each testicle is contained by a fibrous capsule, the tunica albuginea. Anteriorly, the testicle is covered by a thin double-layered sac, the tunica vaginalis, which is the remnant of tissue from the belly cavity that the testicle carries with it as it passes from the abdomen into the scrotum during development. Along the posterior-lateral border of the testis lies the epididymis, which is also partially covered by the tunica vaginalis. The epididymis is the group of convoluted tubes in which the sperm mature and which straighten out to become the vas deferens, the tube that carries sperm from the epididymis to the penis. Other structures within the scrotum include: a) the testicular artery which carries blood to the testicle; b) the pampiniform plexus and testicular vein which carry blood from the testicle back to the body; c) various nerves; and d) lymphatic vessels which help to return fluid that leaks out of the blood vessels into the tissues back to the body.

Table 17-1: Conditions Presenting as Scrotal Masses	
Lesions	**Frequency (%)**
Inflammatory masses	47.8
Hydrocele	23.7
Testicular torsion	9.4
Varicocele	6.8
Spermatocele	4.3
Various cysts	4.0
Malignant tumors	2.2
Hematocele	0.7
Miscellaneous	1.1

Adapted from: *American Journal of Surgery*, vol. 145. Macksood MJ and James RE, "The Scrotal Mass: Cause and Diagnosis," 297-299, 1983, with permission from Excerpta Medica Inc.

Various coverings, or sheaths, derived from the layers of muscle making up the anterior abdominal wall through which the testicle passes, surround the testicle and cord of structures passing to and from the scrotum. These layers of tissue include, from inside out, the internal spermatic fascia, the cremasteric fascia, and the external spermatic fascia. Just beneath the skin of the scrotum is a superficial layer of fascia, the dartos fascia, which contains the dartos muscle. This muscle responds to cold and other stimuli by contracting to draw the testicle nearer to the body.

Any of the structures described above can develop abnormalities which can result in a scrotal mass. Table 17-1 lists some of the more common of these conditions.

EPIDIDYMITIS

As discussed in Chapter 15, epididymitis is an inflammation of the epididymis usually acquired by the spread of bacteria down the vas deferens from the urethra. Patients typically present with pain and swelling in the scrotum. A urinalysis usually reveals evidence of inflammation or infection. Early on, the swelling and tenderness can be localized to the epididymis; however, the distinction between the epididymis and the testicle blurs as the inflammation progresses which makes it more difficult to distinguish epididymitis from torsion. Complications of epididymitis include hydrocele formation, scrotal abscess (i.e., a localized collection of pus), and obstruction of either the epididymis or vas deferens by scarring. Treatment of epididymitis consists primarily of antibiotics and pain control.

ORCHITIS

Orchitis, or inflammation of the testicle, is usually secondary to an extension of a bacterial epididymitis and, therefore, the treatment is identical to that for acute epididymitis. However, isolated orchitis may be the result of a viral infection. Mumps is the most common cause of orchitis. Mumps-related orchitis occurs mostly in post-pubertal males. The patient presents with sudden onset of pain and swelling of the testis, usually occurring four to six days after the appearance of mumps. There are usually no urinary tract complaints, and the urinalysis tends to be normal. In

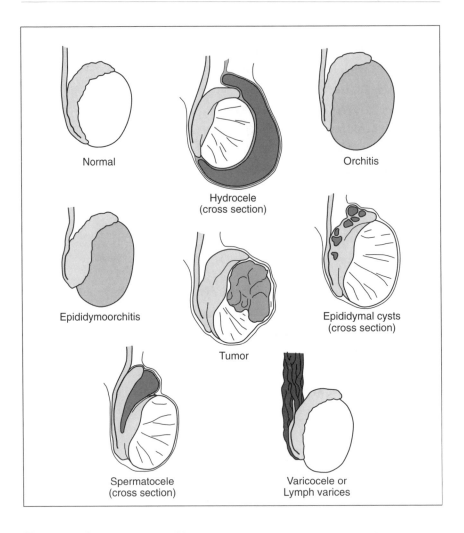

Figure 17-2: Some common conditions that may present as scrotal masses. Reproduced with permission. Paola AS and Khan SA. "Clinical Evaluation of Scrotal Masses: An Overview." HOSPITAL PRACTICE 1989; 24(3):255. ©1989 The McGraw-Hill Companies, Inc. Original illustration by Albert Miller.

two-thirds of cases, only one testicle is involved; the rest of the time, the orchitis is bilateral. Approximately 30 percent of post-pubertal males with mumps will get mumps orchitis, and about 30 percent of these patients will suffer significant testicular damage. In fact, viral orchitis remains the most common cause of acquired testicular failure in the adult. Mumps orchitis will usually resolve on its own in seven to ten days. Treatment consists of bedrest, scrotal elevation, and pain medication until the symptoms improve. The mumps vaccine helps decrease the risk of developing orchitis.

HYDROCELES

There is normally a small amount of fluid between the two layers of the tunica vaginalis. This is usually imperceptible because the amount of fluid produced each day should be equal to the amount of fluid reabsorbed. However, when the amount of fluid produced is greater than the amount reabsorbed, the tunica vaginalis enlarges and becomes palpable as a scrotal mass. A hydrocele is an accumulation of fluid in the tunica vaginalis surrounding the testicle. It is usually painless, but if it achieves a significant size, it can cause discomfort due to its weight. It may also get in the way during walking or make it uncomfortable for a person to wear tight-fitting pants.

On physical examination, hydroceles are usually oval, nontender masses anterior to the testicle that can be transilluminated (i.e., a light can be seen to shine through the fluid of the hydrocele in a dark room). It must be mentioned that 10 percent of testicular tumors may present as a new hydrocele, so if the testicle cannot be completely evaluated on physical examination then an ultrasound of the scrotum is usually performed to confirm the diagnosis.

Hydroceles may be either congenital (present at birth or during infancy; or acquired (i.e., those that develop during adult life).

Congenital Hydroceles

These are usually the result of fluid accumulation in the scrotum from a connection between the belly cavity and the tunica vaginalis, and are present in 6 percent of full-term boys. The resultant scrotal masses may appear and disappear with changes in position. In the infant, this condition may be difficult to differentiate from a hernia. The treatment of an infant hydrocele is usually delayed until after one year of age because spontaneous resolution may occur. After that time, surgical repair via an inguinal approach is usually recommended to drain the hydrocele sac and tie off the connection between the belly cavity and the tunica vaginalis.

Acquired Hydroceles

These are believed to be due to an imbalance between fluid production and reabsorption by the tunica vaginalis. The cause of this imbalance is usually unknown (idiopathic). However, some possible causes include inflammation from epididymitis, tumors, or systemic diseases, such as tuberculosis. Since these hydroceles are usually benign, if they are asymptomatic and the testicle is totally normal, no treatment is usually recommended. However, if the hydrocele is so large that it bothers the person (e.g., discomfort due to size or weight or it gets in the way while walking or when wearing tight pants), treatment is generally indicated.

While needle aspiration has been used for temporary relief, the fluid usually reaccumulates. In addition, needle insertion can result in infection of the hydrocele fluid. Both of these drawbacks make this a less desirable form of treatment for a hydrocele. In the past, certain chemicals have been injected into the tunica vaginalis after aspiration of the fluid in an attempt to cause inflammation and scarring which might prevent fluid reaccumulation; however, this is painful and also runs the risk of infection.

Definitive treatment for healthy, symptomatic patients, usually involves making an incision in the anterolateral aspect of the scrotum to reach the hydrocele sac. The sac is then opened, and the fluid is drained out of the sac. The excess sac surrounding the testicle is then either plicated (sewn together to itself in accordion-like fashion) or cut away from the testicle in an attempt to prevent fluid reaccumulation. The scrotum is then sewn closed.

Some of the risks associated with the surgical repair of a hydrocele include:

1. Infection.
2. Bleeding.
3. Pain, usually temporary, rarely chronic.
4. Damage to other structures (especially the vas deferens which can result in obstruction of the vas and subsequent subfertility).

5. Loss of testicle, since any operation in the scrotum can interfere with the blood supply to the testicle and result in the "death" of the testicle (the testicle then atrophies into a little nubbin of tissue).

6. Recurrence of the hydrocele.

7. Anesthetic risks, such as heart attack, stroke, and death which are small in a healthy person.

TORSION

Torsion occurs when the testicle and spermatic cord twist around a vertical axis. This situation can cause pain and swelling in the testicle, and thus, a painful scrotal mass. If not corrected quickly, torsion can result in death of the testicle. Torsion is discussed in greater detail in Chapter 3.

VARICOCELE

A varicocele is an abnormal dilatation of the veins of the spermatic cord and has been described as feeling like a bag of worms. It can present as a painless scrotal mass, or be discovered in the evaluation of infertility. Varicoceles occur in up to 20 percent of healthy adolescents and young men, and they are rarely detected in boys under 10 years of age. They are found more commonly on the left side. The significance of a varicocele is its association with infertility, with up to 40 percent of subfertile male patients being to found to have a varicocele. A detailed discussion of the evaluation and management of varicoceles is found in Chapter 10.

SPERMATOCELE

The tubes that carry sperm from the testicle to the epididymis are called the efferent ductules. Occasionally, one of these tubes can get blocked, and sperm and fluid collects within it, causing the tube to swell up like a balloon. The result is a spermatocele, a sperm-containing cystic dilatation of an efferent ductule. It is usually located at the head of the epididymis and may be bilateral or multiple. It presents as a painless mass above the testicle, and can usually be felt to be separate from the testicle.

Although most spermatoceles are small (less than 1 cm. in diameter), they may get as big as 8 to 10 cm., which can become uncomfortable. A spermatocele can usually be transilluminated, but in questionable cases, an ultrasound of the scrotum can be used to confirm the diagnosis.

Aspiration of a spermatocele reveals a cloudy, milky fluid containing sperm, just like semen and in contrast to the clear yellow fluid of a hydrocele. However, due to the risk of infection and recurrence, aspiration is *not* recommended. Since any surgery in the scrotum can result in the loss of the testicle or injury to the vas deferens, treatment of spermatoceles is generally not recommended in young men who have yet to have children.

In symptomatic men who no longer desire children, definitive treatment consists of surgical removal of the spermatocele. This operation is called spermatocelectomy. An incision is made in the anterolateral aspect of the affected side of the scrotum, and dissection is continued down to the testicle. The spermatocele is dissected from the surrounding structures, and its connection to the testicle is tied off. The spermatocele is then removed. The patient usually goes home a few hours after surgery. In patients with multiple spermatoceles, the entire epididymis may have to be removed as well. Some risks of spermatocelectomy include infection, bleeding, and temporary or chronic pain. Despite the removal of the spermatocele, other spermatoceles may develop. Additional (but rare) risks include hydrocele formation, loss of testicle, obstruction of the vas deferens, and the risks of anesthesia (which include heart attack, stroke, and death).

CYSTS

Occasionally, the tubes of the epididymis can balloon out to form cystic cavities that may present as painless scrotal masses, or which are observed on an ultrasound of the scrotum being performed for other reasons. These epididymal cysts can usually be felt to be separate from the testicle; however, in equivocal cases, ultrasound can confirm the diagnosis. Since epididymal cysts are usually asymptomatic and of no consequence, treatment is not required unless they become large and cause problems due to their size. In these rare instances, surgical removal of the cysts or of the entire epididymis may be necessary.

TESTICULAR TUMORS

It must be stressed that a scrotal mass felt to be within the testicle itself should be considered to be a testicular cancer until proven otherwise, and it mandates prompt surgical exploration through an inguinal incision. Testicular cancers typically present as a painless lump in the scrotum of a young man between the ages of 18 and 40. Tumors occur 11 times more frequently in undescended testicles than in normally descended ones, and 50 times more frequently in undescended testes that were discovered in the abdomen. They are very rare in men of African descent.

Although the person with a testicular tumor usually complains of incidentally noting a painless scrotal lump, he may also have experienced a heavy sensation or a dull ache in the scrotum or lower abdomen, due to the weight of the mass. Occasionally, testicular tumors can present with sudden, severe pain secondary to rapid growth from bleeding within the tumor. Physical examination usually reveals a firm, nontender mass arising from the testicle. Up to 10 percent of testis cancers will initially present with either a hydrocele or symptoms consistent with epididymitis. Again, in equivocal cases, or those in which the testicle cannot be completely palpated, scrotal ultrasound may help clarify the problem.

Benign testicular tumors are rare (less than 1 percent). Therefore, intratesticular masses should be considered malignant until a pathologic diagnosis proves otherwise. Adequate treatment of a mass believed to be a testicular cancer involves removing the affected testicle and spermatic cord through an inguinal incision. A detailed discussion of testicular cancer is located in Chapter 24.

HEMATOCELE/TRAUMA

A hematocele is a collection of blood in the tunica vaginalis which is most commonly due to trauma. These patients present with pain and swelling following trauma to the scrotum. One important problem in scrotal trauma is deciding whether the testicular capsule has remained intact, a condition known as scrotal contusion, or if it has been ruptured, a condition known as testicular fracture. Ultrasound can be helpful since testicular fracture is almost always associated with a hematocele. Scrotal contusions can be managed conservatively with ice packs and pain medication until the pain and swelling resolves, but testicular fracture requires immediate surgical exploration to drain the hematocele and repair the injury to the testicular capsule so that the injured testicle is not lost.

INGUINAL HERNIA

An inguinal hernia is a result of a weakness in the muscles that make up the abdominal wall. The intestines can push out through this weak area and are felt as a bulge in the inguinal or groin region. If these loops of bowel push their way into the scrotum, an inguinal hernia can present as a scrotal mass in adults. In infants, sometimes the canal that the testicle forms when it goes from the belly cavity into the scrotum does not close off, and the intestines can push down into this canal forming a hernia as well. These hernias occur in 3 to 5 percent of full-term infants, are nine times more common in males than females, and are located more commonly on the right side.

The danger of inguinal hernias is that when the piece of intestine pushes through the hole, or weakness, in the abdominal wall, it might have its blood supply compromised. This condition, known as strangulation of the hernia, is a surgical emergency that can result in "death" of the involved piece of intestine —a life-threatening situation. Therefore, due to the risks associated with complications of hernias, it is usually recommended to repair a hernia electively when it is diagnosed rather than risk developing a complication, such as strangulation, which requires surgical management under emergent conditions. Since approximately 15 percent of inguinal hernias in infants are bilateral, it is usually recommended that, in infants up to two years of age who undergo a hernia repair, the other inguinal area be explored under the same anesthesia in case a small hernia is present on that side, too.

PARATESTICULAR TUMORS

Paratesticular tumors are masses that arise from structures outside the testicle but within the scrotum. They account for less than 10 percent of all intrascrotal tumors. These rare tumors are most commonly benign (for example, they are often lipomas, or benign tumors of fat cells). However, malignant tumors of the spermatic cord and tunica vaginalis can occur. Paratesticular masses can usually be felt as separate from the testicle, but again, in equivocal cases, ultrasound can be helpful.

In general, most extratesticular masses are cystic and benign, while most intratesticular lesions are solid and malignant. Any extratesticular masses suspicious for cancer may require surgical removal of the testis and spermatic cord via an inguinal approach for pathologic diagnosis.

POLYORCHIDISM

During the development of the embryo, the tissue destined to become a testicle can sometimes split which will result in an extra testicle developing on one side, so that the person is born with more than the usual two testicles. This harmless condition is known as *polyorchidism*, and tends to present as a painless scrotal mass. The ipsilateral testicles share the same blood supply, but each testicle usually has its own epididymis and vas deferens, which can be palpated on physical examination. Therefore, in patients presenting with a solid extratesticular mass and two vasa deferentia on the same side, the diagnosis of polyorchidism is usually considered.

SCROTAL EDEMA

Excess fluid retained by the body can accumulate in the lower extremities, including the scrotum. This excess fluid, or edema, can cause the scrotal sac to swell, making it appear as though the person has a scrotal mass. The physical examination is otherwise normal. Some conditions that can result in scrotal edema include congestive heart failure, kidney failure, or obstruction to lymphatic flow from prior surgery, radiation treatments, cancer, or inflammatory processes (e.g., parasitic diseases, syphilis, or tuberculosis). A conservative treatment approach is usually recommended, which involves elevation of the scrotum on towels (to encourage fluid drainage by gravity) and appropriate management of the underlying medical problem.

Other lesions involving the scrotal skin include sebaceous cysts, fungal infections, and skin cancers. These are usually distinguishable from intrascrotal masses on physical examination, and any questionable lesions usually require further evaluation and management by a dermatologist.

Most people and physicians hear "scrotal mass" and think: *cancer*. In a way this is good, because it usually leads the patient to promptly seek medical attention. Extratesticular scrotal masses tend to outnumber intratesticular ones, which is also good because most intratesticular lesions are malignant and most extratesticular masses are benign. The patient's history helps the physician narrow down the possible causes of a scrotal mass. Of special importance in the history is whether or not the mass is painful. A physical examination, with the help of transillumination, will usually help determine if the mass is intratesticular or extratesticular, and whether it's solid or cystic. A urinalysis can sometimes be helpful in cases of possible infection (e.g., epididymitis). In equivocal cases, a scrotal ultrasound may also be of benefit to demonstrate the location of the lesion. The lesson to learn is that if you feel something extra or strange in the scrotum, take the family jewels in for a check-up to be sure nothing bad is going on.

References

1. Ellis H: *Clinical Anatomy*, 6th ed. Oxford: Blackwell Scientific Publications, 1977.
2. Hall-Craggs ECB: *Anatomy as a Basis for Clinical Medicine*, Baltimore - Munich: Urban and Schwarzenberg, 1985.
3. Macfarlane MT: *Urology for the House Officer*, 2nd ed. Baltimore: Williams and Wilkins, 1995.
4. Macksood MJ and James RE: "The Scrotal Mass: Cause and Diagnosis." *Am J Surg* 1983, 145(2):297-299.
5. Paola AS and Khan SA: "Clinical Evaluation of Scrotal Masses: An Overview." *Hospital Practice* (Off Ed) 1989, 24(3):255-258, 259-264.

CHAPTER 18

HEMATURIA

Blood in the urine is known as *hematuria*. When the quantity of blood is large, it can be seen by the naked eye as reddish discoloration of the urine; a condition known as *gross hematuria*. A small amount of blood in the urine, detectable only with a microscope, is called *microscopic hematuria*. Hematuria can be a manifestation of many urinary tract diseases. In this chapter, the discussion will be limited to the evaluation of patients with this problem. Some of the common causes of hematuria are discussed in greater detail in other parts of this book.

Hematuria, whether gross or microscopic, is worrisome to both the patient and the physician because it may be a sign of urinary tract cancer. In one study of patients with gross hematuria, tumors were found in approximately 22 percent of patients. The risk of finding a cancer in patients with microscopic hematuria has been reported to be between 2 and 13 percent. Some other common causes of hematuria include: infection, stones, benign prostatic hyperplasia, trauma, sickle cell disease, medical kidney diseases (glomerulonephritis), tuberculosis, problems with clotting factors in the blood, exercise (for instance, jogging), and vascular disease. It is important to note that bleeding in the urinary tract can be intermittent; however, the episodic nature of the problem and the absence of other symptoms should not deter the patient from proceeding with an evaluation.

As in the evaluation of any medical problem, an accurate diagnosis is based on a thorough history and physical examination and various laboratory and special studies.

HISTORY

Physicians use the history obtained from a patient to help figure out the source of the bleeding. Some aspects of the patient's history which help to classify hematuria include timing, associated symptoms, and age.

Blood noted at the start of voiding, known as *initial hematuria*, is usually from the penile part of the urethra. Blood noted just at the end of urination, *terminal hematuria*, is usually associated with bleeding from the prostate or the area where the prostate meets the bladder, called the bladder neck. Blood noted throughout urination, *total hematuria*, usually indicates bleeding at or above the level of the bladder.

Irritative voiding symptoms (i.e., frequency, urgency, or dysuria) may point to a urinary tract infection or bladder tumor. Back pain localized to one side makes one suspect a kidney stone. A history of recent trauma could be responsible for the blood. Drugs that "thin" the blood (e.g., Coumadin, aspirin, or ibuprofen) may make a person bleed more easily, but one must be careful not to blame the bleeding on the medication. Abnormal lesions in the urinary tract may be unmasked at an earlier stage in patients on these medications. A history of tobacco use is often found in patients with bladder tumors. Hematuria in black patients should also raise the suspicion of sickle cell disease.

The age and sex of a person with hematuria are also somewhat helpful when considering a diagnosis. Table 18-1 shows the most common causes of hematuria, categorized by age and sex. Although the risk of significant lesions increases after age 40, it must be remembered that statistics are useful for the general population rather than for individuals. Therefore, patients should not be lulled into a false sense of security.

Table 18-1: The Most Common Causes of Hematuria by Age and Sex	
Age (years)/Sex	**Common Causes**
0 - 20/males & females	Acute glomerulonephritis
	Acute urinary tract infection
	Urinary tract anomalies present at birth which cause obstruction to urine flow
	Elevated calcium levels in the urine
20 - 40/males & females	Acute urinary tract infection
	Stones
	Bladder tumor
40 - 60/males	Bladder tumor
	Stones
	Acute urinary tract infection
40 - 60/females	Acute urinary tract infection
	Stones
	Bladder tumor
> 60/males	Benign prostatic hyperplasia
	Bladder tumor
	Acute urinary tract infection
> 60/females	Bladder tumor
	Acute urinary tract infection

From: Gillenwater JY, *et al.*, *Adult and Pediatric Urology*, 3rd ed. St. Louis: Mosby, 1996, p. 657.

PHYSICAL EXAMINATION

Although the physical exam tends to be unremarkable in most patients exhibiting hematuria, it can sometimes shed light on the source of the bleeding. For example, the presence of high blood pressure, otherwise known as *hypertension*, may signal a medical cause of the bleeding. Fever suggests an infectious etiology, although some kidney cancers can also cause low-grade fevers. A mass found on the abdominal exam may suggest a kidney tumor. Examination of the genitalia may also reveal the source of the hematuria, for example urethral warts near the meatus; a foreign body in the urethra; or prostate abnormalities, such as prostatitis, prostate cancer, or benign prostatic hyperplasia.

LABORATORY OR SPECIAL STUDIES

Red urine doesn't always mean blood. Pigmenturia is a reddish discoloration of the urine caused by something other than blood, and can be due to various foods, drugs, or chemicals. A urinalysis will confirm the presence of a significant amount of blood in the urine (i.e., more than 3 to 5 red blood cells seen consistently with a high power microscope), and it will also distinguish hematuria from pigmenturia. When hematuria is confirmed on urinalysis, a urine culture is usually performed to rule out a urinary tract infection (UTI). In the case of a UTI, it is recommended to repeat the urinalysis after the infection has been treated, since a UTI may occur coincidentally with another cause of hematuria, such as a stone or a tumor. If the hematuria persists after treatment of the infection, or if no infection is documented, further evaluation is indicated.

Various blood tests are usually done in patients with hematuria. First of all, tests that evaluate kidney function—especially a serum creatinine—are important, since some of the dyes used in x-ray studies can adversely affect renal function. Complete blood counts (CBC) can give an idea as to the severity of the blood loss. In cases of gross hematuria, the person's clotting factors are evaluated to check for coagulopathies. Finally, an evaluation for sickle cell disease is recommended for all black patients with hematuria.

In patients with hematuria and normal kidney function, an intravenous pyelogram (IVP) is the best test to search for abnormalities in the kidneys and ureters (the tubes that carry urine from the kidneys to the bladder). During an IVP, dye which is injected into an arm vein gets filtered by the kidney, and x-rays are taken to visualize the kidneys, ureters, and bladder. This test can reveal kidney stones, tumors, obstruction to urine flow, or other problems in the upper urinary tract (the kidneys and ureter).

There are several risks associated with IVP. The procedure often has vasomotor effects—approximately 50 percent of patients experience a feeling of warmth, nausea or vomiting, or a metallic taste, which are of no clinical significance. Approximately 5 percent of patients have allergic reactions, and show mild to moderate redness, itching, or hives that usually respond to benadryl. However, in approximately 1 in 1000 patients, respiratory problems can occur as a result of IVP, and these patients require epinephrine and possibly cardiopulmonary resuscitation (CPR).

The risk of death from an IVP is approximately 1 in 40,000 to 1 in 75,000. Some newer dyes that are associated with a lower risk of allergic reactions are used in patients with a history of allergic reactions to intravenous dyes or of an allergy to iodine-containing materials. In cases where the risk of an allergic reaction is high, the patient may be started on steroids four to five days before the IVP to try to decrease the risk of an allergic reaction.

The dye used to help visualize the kidneys during an IVP can occasionally impair kidney function and, in rare instances, lead to renal failure. In patients with normal renal function, the risk of this problem is low (i.e., approximately 0.8%). Pre-existing renal insufficiency is the most important risk factor for renal failure after contrast administration; therefore, the doctor will usually check a person's kidney function by obtaining a blood test, called a serum creatinine level, before performing an IVP. If the creatinine level is less than 2 mg/dL in non-diabetics (and less than 1.5 mg/dL in patients with diabetes mellitus), the risk of renal failure after IVP is relatively low.

A final risk of IVP is to the cardiovascular system. Rarely, the administration of dye can lead to a stress on the heart and will precipitate fluid overload, a situation known as *congestive heart failure*.

Any abnormalities found on IVP will require further evaluation which depends on the location and type of abnormality found. For example, a mass in the kidney will require further evaluation with either an ultrasound or CT scan. Any incomplete filling of the urinary tubes from the kidney to the bladder raises the question of tumor, stone, or clot, and requires cystoscopy and retrograde pyelography, a procedure where a small telescope is passed from the penis through the urethra into the bladder and dye is injected up the ureters from the bladder under anesthesia. Further evaluation of these filling defects may require ureteroscopy, which involves passing a very narrow telescope up the urethra, bladder and ureter to directly visualize any abnormality found in the upper urinary tract.

If the IVP is normal, examination of the bladder and urethra still needs to be carried out since an IVP is not sensitive enough to adequately evaluate the bladder or urethra. In cystoscopy, the patient is placed on the table with his legs up in stirrups, and his penis and scrotal area are cleaned. An anesthetic jelly is inserted into the penis via the urethral meatus to help decrease the discomfort from the cystoscope. The cystoscope is then inserted into the urethra and advanced into the bladder, and visual examination of the urethra and bladder is carried out. Some fluid is usually taken from the bladder and sent to the laboratory to search for the presence of cancerous cells, a test known as cytology.

Some risks of cystoscopy include infection, bleeding or blood-spotting of underwear for a short time after the procedure, discomfort (especially during passage of the cystoscope through the prostatic urethra), burning on urination for one or two days after the procedure, urethral stricture (i.e., scar formation in the urethra), and urinary retention (the inability to urinate due to prostatic swelling after the procedure).

In patients with poor renal function, as evidenced by a serum creatinine greater than 2 mg/dL (or greater than 1.5 mg/dL in patients with diabetes mellitus), an IVP can cause further damage to the kidneys. In these cases, the recommended evaluation is an ultrasound of the kidneys (to rule out a renal mass), followed by cystoscopy and retrograde pyelogram in the operating room.

If the initial urologic work-up of hematuria, including IVP, cystoscopy, and cytology, doesn't reveal an obvious source of the blood, the risk of developing a significant or life-threatening lesion is low (under 1 percent). The source of the hematuria remains unknown in approximately 25 percent of patients evaluated for hematuria with the these studies. More in-depth examination with other studies may reveal a source, but these are rarely significant lesions. Although hematuria cannot occur without a cause, even after in-depth evaluations, 5 to 10 percent of patients will have no obvious source. The diagnosis of idiopathic hematuria, however, remains one of exclusion. It is suggested that hematuria patients with a negative initial work-up have a urine specimen sent for urinalysis and cytology every six to twelve months for two to three years unless gross hematuria recurs or new symptoms develop, just to make sure that nothing is missed.

The problem of hematuria in children less than 16 years old differs slightly. Since UTIs and anatomical abnormalities are the most common urologic causes of hematuria in children, the history, physical examination, urinalysis, culture and blood work to evaluate renal function are part of the recommended initial work-up of hematuria in children. After this, children believed to have a medical problem causing their hematuria, such as glomerulonephritis, are usually referred to a nephrologist—a doctor who specializes in medical diseases that affect the kidney. If, however, the cause of the hematuria is believed to be urologic, the recommended work-up includes: 1) an IVP or renal ultrasound to evaluate the upper tracts, and 2) a voiding cystourethrogram (VCUG) to search for abnormalities in the bladder and urethra.

A VCUG is an x-ray study in which dye is injected up the urethra into the bladder and pictures are taken before, during, and after urinating. Any abnormalities found on these studies will require further evaluation and management. If these studies are unremarkable, a search for elevated levels of calcium in the urine is also considered, since hypercalciuria has been reported to cause hematuria in children.

The need for cystoscopy in the evaluation of hematuria in children is controversial. On the one hand, one of the phrases that all physicians try to remember, especially when dealing with children, is *primum non nocere* –that is, first do no harm. On the other hand, one doesn't want to miss anything. In the presence of gross hematuria, cystoscopy is indicated. In other instances, cystoscopy is usually not recommended since it appears to add little information in these children; however, when to perform imaging and cystoscopy in a child with hematuria is a question that, ultimately, must be answered by the urologist. Today, if parents have questions or want a second opinion regarding further management of their child, they can usually be referred to a pediatric urologist.

Blood in the urine is a red flag–a warning of potential problems. The blood may originate from anywhere in the urinary tract, and whether the hematuria is gross or microscopic, it should be evaluated.

References

1. Gillenwater JY, Grayhack JT, Howards SS, and Duckett JW (eds.): *Adult and Pediatric Urology*, 3rd ed. St. Louis: Mosby, 1996.
2. Kaplan GW: "Hematuria in Children." *AUA Update Series* 1985, vol. 4, lesson 4.
3. Macfarlane MT: *Urology for the House Officer*, 2nd ed. Baltimore: Williams and Wilkins, 1995.
4. Mariani AJ: "The Evaluation of Adult Hematuria." *AUA Update Series* 1989, vol. 8, lesson 4.
5. Mariani AJ: "The Evaluation of Adult Hematuria: A Clinical Update." *AUA Update Series* 1998; vol. 17, lesson 24.
6. Noe HN: "Hematuria in Children." *AUA Update Series* 1997; vol. 16, lesson 34.

CHAPTER 19

KIDNEY STONES

Kidney stones can be a real pain in the... back. You're cruising along in life without a care, and, from out of the blue, you notice a nagging pain on one side of your back. The pain builds in intensity until it's possibly the worst pain of your life. You get nauseated and vomit until it feels like you're heaving your guts out. Then, you either call your doctor, whose secretary can only squeeze you in next week, or go to the hospital looking as if you're trying out for a part in "ER."

Most patients who have had a kidney stone want to know why stones form. It's usually because these patients don't drink enough water. The chemicals that make up stones get excreted into the urine as part of the body's normal metabolic processes. In order for these chemicals to join together and form a crystal, which merges with other crystals to form a stone, they must be highly concentrated in the urine, a condition known as supersaturation. If supersaturation does not exist, a stone cannot form. A high intake of water dilutes the chemicals in the urine and, thus, may prevent supersaturation. This is one reason why doctors tell stone patients to drink plenty of fluids. However, urine may become supersaturated after meals, especially after those that contain large amounts of stone constituents, such as calcium or oxalate. In addition, urine can become supersaturated during sleep, permitting stone development and growth. Another important aspect of stone formation is the presence in the urine of chemicals that inhibit crystal growth. Chemicals known to inhibit calcium stone formation include citrate and magnesium. Some people who don't form stones may have a higher urinary concentration of these inhibitors than do those who tend to form stones. The combination of urinary supersaturation and decreased inhibition may permit the development of small crystals in the urine, but in order for a stone to form, these crystals also must be held in the kidney long enough for them to grow to a size that makes them clinically significant.

This is called particle retention. One theory is that stone-formers have some minimal abnormality in the kidney that allows the crystals to stick to the walls lining the kidney long enough for them to grow into a stone.

The incidence of stone disease is approximately one to three per 1000 persons per year, depending on what part of the country you live in. Climate, geography, and diet are important factors in stone development. For example, stones are more common in the southern part of the United States, possibly due to the warmer climate in the South. A high salt intake has been shown to increase urinary calcium excretion and decrease urinary citrate excretion, and thus, it is a risk factor for calcium stone formation. A high protein diet has also been associated with an increased risk of developing certain stones. Excessive sweating, as can occur in warmer climates or during summer months, can result in a decreased urine volume, and therefore, an increase in the urinary concentration of calcium and other stone constituents predisposing to stone formation. Some studies have attempted to search for an association between the consumption of carbonated beverages or tea and stone formation, but no definite conclusions have been reached yet. Some disease processes are also associated with an increased risk of stone formation (e.g., gout, hyperparathyroidism, sarcoidosis, and certain cancers).

There are four basic types of stones based on their predominant chemical composition: calcium stones, infections stones, uric acid stones, and cystine stones. Calcium stones are usually composed of calcium oxalate or calcium phosphate. They account for approximately 70 to 80 percent of all stone disease in the United States. Infection stones are usually made up of magnesium, ammonium, and phosphate, which are associated with urinary tract infections. Infection stones account for approximately 15 percent of stone disease. Uric acid stones are present in 5 to 10 percent of stone formers. Cystine stones make up 1 to 6 percent of stone patients.

Calcium oxalate is the most common component of urinary tract stones. Calcium phosphate is the second most common component, and it is usually found in association with calcium oxalate. Studies have shown that the most important factors of calcium stone formation, in order of importance, include: 1) decreased urine volumes; 2) increased urinary oxalate excretion; 3) alkaline urine (i.e., high urine pH); 4) increased urinary uric acid excretion (in fact, up to 20 percent of calcium stone formers have this problem which is known as hyperuricosuria); 5) decreased amounts of inhibitors in the urine; and 6) increased urinary calcium excretion. These factors are all taken into account when discussing measures to prevent the formation of calcium stones.

Infection stones are made up of magnesium ammonium phosphate and occur in the highly alkaline urine which results from infection with certain types of bacteria. The high pH (greater than 7.2) reduces the solubility of magnesium ammonium phosphate in the urine, so it crystallizes and forms a stone. Foreign bodies, such as catheters, or neurologic problems which involve the bladder and prevent its normal emptying, are risk factors for infection stones.

Uric acid stones form in the setting of low urine volume, an acid urine (pH less than 6.0), and high levels of uric acid in the urine (i.e., hyperuricosuria). Uric acid is a product of protein metabolism. Uric acid stones are difficult to see on plain x-rays (that is, they are radiolucent), unlike calcium or infection stones which usually show up very well as whitish objects on a dark background of the x-ray film (they are radiopaque). Some drugs, including aspirin compounds and thiazide diuretics (the classic "water pills" used to treat high blood pressure) result in increased urinary excretion of uric acid. Some cancers and their treatment can result in rapid cell turnover, and certain metabolic birth defects can also result in increased production of uric acid which predisposes to uric acid stone formation.

Cystinuria is an inherited defect in the kidney's ability to reabsorb cystine and certain other amino acids. Cystine stones result from increased concentrations of cystine in an acidic urine. A family history of significant stone disease can usually be elicited in these patients.

There are other more rare types of stones, including some which result when certain medications crystallize in the urine (e.g., triamterene and sulfa drugs). Although the initial evaluation and management of most urinary tract stones is basically the same, the following discussion of stone management will deal mainly with the more common types of stones.

The patient with a kidney stone typically presents with back pain just beneath the lowest rib on either side (i.e., flank area), depending on which side the stone is on. The pain can start out as a dull ache, but can increase in intensity to become unbearable. The pain may be felt in the upper or lower abdomen and may even radiate into the testicle on the affected side, since the kidney and testicle share a similar nerve supply. The pain may be intermittent, but unlike back pain from arthritis or other musculoskeletal origin, stone pain doesn't improve with changes in position.

As the stone moves into the upper or middle part of the ureter, the pain is usually felt in the lower abdomen on the side of the stone. As the stone nears the bladder, patients may not only experience flank pain but may also feel the urge to void more frequently. This is because the stone irritates the bladder as it attempts to pass. Pain from a stone occurs when the stone blocks the ureter resulting in rapid distention of the kidney and ureter from retained urine (see Figure 19-1). This rapid swelling is felt as flank pain. In addition to this pain, the ureter then tries to push the stone out by increasing the strength of its contractions and subsequently goes into spasm causing more pain, just like spasms in any muscle. The term renal colic is used to describe the "classic" pain caused by stones. The pain can sometimes be so severe as to cause nausea and vomiting. Patients may also develop gross hematuria if the stone irritates the lining of the urinary tract. Low grade fever may be noted, but a high fever suggests infection.

Unless kidney stones cause some degree of obstruction, they may not be symptomatic. In fact, some patients are found to have kidney stones when being evaluated for other problems and never had any symptoms related to the kidney stone.

Various lab tests and special studies are used to evaluate patients suspected of having a kidney stone. In most cases, a urinalysis will demonstrate some degree of hematuria, but approximately 10 percent of patients with stones don't have hematuria. A urine culture is usually performed to rule out infection. A blood creatinine level is done to check kidney function since the dyes used in IVP (see following page) or other x-ray studies can worsen already impaired renal function (normal serum creatinine is less than 1.5 mg/dL, but unless the patient has diabetes, anything less than 2.0 mg/dL is usually considered acceptable for dye administration).

A plain x-ray of the abdomen including the kidney, ureter, and bladder areas, known as a KUB, is used to search for stones. In fact, 90 percent of stones will be seen on a KUB. As mentioned, uric acid stones are radiolucent

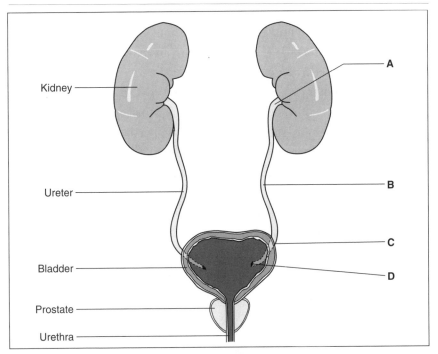

Figure 19-1: *Kidneys, ureters, and bladder and points of narrowing where stones usually get stuck: A) ureteropelvic junction; B) where the ureter crosses over blood vessels in the pelvis; C) ureterovesical junction where the ureter meets the bladder; and D) intramural ureter where the ureter passes through the bladder muscle.*

and may not be seen on plain x-rays. A word of caution: pregnant women should not be exposed to x-rays. Therefore, a pregnant woman believed to have a kidney stone should undergo an ultrasound examination instead.

An intravenous pyelogram (IVP) is a radiographic study in which dye injected into a vein is filtered and concentrated by the kidneys (see Chapter 18). Then, pictures of the kidneys, ureters, and bladder are taken. This test usually demonstrates the size and location of stones as well as the degree of obstruction. Even radiolucent stones will usually be seen on IVP. Sometimes, however, small, non-obstructing stones may not be seen on IVP. The risks of IVP are discussed in Chapter 18.

In patients whose kidney function is so poor that dye administration is contraindicated, studies that are sometimes used to demonstrate the presence of a stone include KUB, ultrasound of the kidneys, CT scan of the abdomen without contrast, and cystoscopy with retrograde pyelogram (see Chapter 18), but these instances are rare.

Once a stone is diagnosed, the first important step in management is to control the pain. There are various prescription pain medications that make the patient feel much better and allow him to tolerate the stone until definitive treatment is carried out. If the patient's pain cannot be controlled, he is usually admitted to the hospital for monitoring, more powerful pain medication, and possibly surgery if his pain still persists. Other indications to admit stone patients to the hospital include: 1) high fever (greater than 101° F) which requires intravenous antibiotics to treat possible infection, since infection in the presence of obstruction from a stone can severely damage the kidney; 2) severe dehydration from nausea and vomiting which requires the administration of intravenous fluids; and 3) an obstructed solitary kidney.

Immediate care of the stone patient depends on the size of the stone which helps determine the likelihood that it will pass spontaneously, any complicating medical problems (e.g., solitary kidney), and complications related to the stone itself, such as high grade obstruction or infection. The chance that a stone less than 5 mm. in diameter will pass spontaneously is approximately 80 to 98 percent. Stones 5 to 8 mm. in size have a 50 percent chance of passing spontaneously, while stones greater than 8 to 10 mm. in diameter are unlikely to pass spontaneously.

There are several different treatment options for kidney and ureteral stones. Treatments are usually recommended based on the size and the location of the stone.

WATCHFUL WAITING

Figure 19-1 shows the most common sites where stones "hang up" during passage: 1) the ureteropelvic junction where the kidney meets the ureter; 2) where the ureter crosses over blood vessels in the pelvis; 3) where the ureter meets the bladder; and 4) at the end of the ureter as it passes through the bladder muscle. It is at these sites of narrowing where stones most commonly get caught and obstruct the ureter causing distention of the ureter with resultant renal colic. Approximately 50 percent of symptomatic stones will pass spontaneously; the others will require surgical intervention.

Stones less than 5 mm. in diameter have up to a 98 percent chance of passing spontaneously, and are generally given one month to pass, as long as the patient is comfortable. The patient is asked to drink about 1 gallon of fluid per day, half of which should be water, to try to flush out the stone. He is also asked to strain all urine in an effort to catch any stone that passes, and to save any stones that pass for analysis. Oral medications are given for pain control. If the patient fails to pass the stone by the follow-up visit, other treatment options can be pursued.

Stones larger than 8 mm. in diameter are unlikely to pass on their own, so watchful waiting is usually not recommended. With regard to stones 5 to 8 mm. in size, treatment usually depends on stone location. If the stone has already made it into the lower part of the ureter, a trial of watchful waiting may be worthwhile. However, if the stone is in the kidney or upper ureter, the decision may depend on the patient's symptoms.

Sometimes patients can't or won't wait the recommended time to pass the stone on their own. For example, airplane pilots are grounded until their stone is taken care of. In addition, occasionally the great pain from renal colic cannot be controlled with oral medication. Other indications for early surgical intervention in patients with kidney stones include: 1) high grade obstruction from the stone (if it is not taken care of within a few weeks, it can result in significant damage to the kidney); 2) persistent infection despite antibiotics; 3) uncontrollable pain; and 4) impairment of renal function or solitary kidney.

MEDICAL THERAPY TO DISSOLVE STONES

Uric acid and cystine are very soluble in alkaline solutions. Occasionally, an attempt can be made to dissolve uric acid or cystine stones by using medication to make the urine alkaline (i.e., pH greater than 6.5 for uric acid stones or greater than 7.5 for cystine stones). Sodium bicarbonate or potassium citrate can be used to achieve this goal. One problem is that it may take several weeks or even months to dissolve a large stone completely using this treatment option. In fact, in cases of larger uric acid or cystine stones, treatments that fragment the stones may be used first, and then, dissolution therapy can be used to treat the residual smaller fragments.

Another significant problem with dissolution therapy is that calcium stones account for 70 to 80 percent of all stones, and, to date, a medication to dissolve calcium stones has not been found.

ENDOSCOPIC TREATMENT

Cystoscopy/Ureteral Stent Placement

Cystoscopy involves the passage of a telescopic instrument up the urethra into the bladder under anesthesia. A stent (which is a hollow tube about 24 to 28 cm. long, about as big around as the refill of a Bic pen and coiled at both ends) is passed up the ureter through the cystoscope and is positioned so that one end is located in the kidney and the other end is in the bladder. Since it is hollow, urine can pass through the stent to bypass any obstruction from a stone. This relieves the dilatation of the ureter and can resolve renal colic. This is basically a temporary procedure to relieve significant obstruction and pain from a stone until definitive treatment can be carried out. Cystoscopy and stent placement can also be used in conjunction with other treatment options.

Risks of this procedure include: infection, bleeding, pain, urethral stricture (i.e., scar tissue in the urethra), failure to place the stent due to obstruction from the stone, perforation of the ureter during stent placement (very rare), stent irritation, and anesthetic risks. Stent irritation is usually felt as a need to urinate more frequently or a discomfort in the lower abdomen or flank area at the end of voiding. However, at times stent irritation can be so significant that some patients have said that the pain from the stent was worse than their stone pain.

Once the stone is taken care of, the stent needs to be removed. In the past, stent removal required cystoscopy, but this is no longer necessary. Now, stents come with strings attached. The string can be brought out through the patient's urethral meatus and is taped to his penis until the stent is no longer needed. Then, the stent is removed by the patient by pulling on the string.

Cystoscopy/Ureteroscopy/Stone Removal

Ureteroscopy involves the passage of a telescopic instrument up the urethra into the bladder and then up the ureter to directly visualize the stone. At this point, various wire graspers, or baskets (miniature instruments which can be passed through the ureteroscope to grab or ensnare the stone) can be used to pull out the stone. If the stone is too large to remove with graspers or baskets, it can be fragmented into smaller pieces by various instruments called lithotripters which can be passed through the ureteroscope. Then, the smaller fragments can usually be removed with either graspers or baskets.

Three types of endoscopic lithotripters may be used: 1) electrohydraulic lithotripters, which use shock waves generated by a miniature spark plug to fragment the stone; 2) ultrasonic lithotripters, which use sonic waves generated by vibration to grind the stone into smaller pieces; and 3) laser lithotripters, which uses a laser beam to fragment the stone. All of these methods are highly successful at fragmenting stones. After the fragments are removed, a ureteral stent is usually left in place for a few days until the ureteral swelling from surgery resolves. Again, in most cases, a stent with an attached string can be placed to avoid having to perform cystoscopy to remove the stent. Cystoscopy/ureteroscopy and stone removal usually lasts about 45 minutes to one hour, and patients usually go home the same day or the following morning with antibiotics and pain medication.

Risks of these procedures include: infection, bleeding, pain, urethral stricture, bladder perforation, failure to perform ureteroscopy (2 percent), ureteral injury (4 to 10 percent) which is usually managed with stent placement for 3 to 6 weeks, significant injury to the ureter requiring open surgery to repair (0.5 percent), ureteral stricture (0.5 to 11 percent), failure to fragment the stone, residual stone fragments which might require further treatment, failure to place a ureteral stent, stent irritation, and anesthetic risk.

Percutaneous Nephrostolithotripsy

Percutaneous nephrostolithotripsy (PNL) is a type of endoscopic treatment for kidney stones. In this procedure, a needle is inserted through the patient's back into the affected kidney under anesthesia. Using dilators passed over a guide wire, a track about 7 to 10 mm. in diameter is made which allows the passage of a telescopic instrument, called a nephroscope, into the kidney to directly visualize the stone. Then, using one of the various lithotripters described above, the stone is fragmented into pieces small enough to be removed with graspers or baskets. The operation usually takes from one to two hours, depending on the size of the stone. A drainage tube, called a nephrostomy tube, is placed in the kidney at the end of the procedure. It is brought out through the flank and hooked up to a drainage bag that attaches to the patient's leg. The nephrostomy tube is left in place until it is confirmed that no significant stone fragments remain.

Since this procedure is usually performed on larger stones (stones greater than 2.5 cm. in diameter), residual fragments can be found on follow-up visits, and these patients may require additional procedures, such as repeat PNL or extracorporeal shock wave lithotripsy (see below), to become stone free. Patients are usually discharged with antibiotics and pain medication one to two days after surgery depending on how the operation goes.

Risks of PNL include infection, bleeding, the need for transfusion (approximately 10 percent), pain, residual stone fragments, need for open surgery to stop bleeding (rare), damage to adjacent structures, perforation of the kidney or ureter which is usually just treated with prolonged nephrostomy tube drainage, lung injury (0.1 to 1 percent), heart attack, and death (0.04 to 0.2 percent).

Extracorporeal Shock Wave Lithotripsy (ESWL)

ESWL is a non-invasive method of treating urinary tract stones by generating shock waves outside the body and focusing them on stones to fragment them into pieces small enough to pass spontaneously. The basic mechanism of stone fragmentation is that shock waves generated outside the body can be transmitted through water and then pass through the patient's body to get to the stone. X-rays are used to aim the shock waves at the stone. Repeated shock waves lead to cracks at weak points in the stone and its eventual fragmentation. Initially, these shock waves were generated in a bathtub, and although the "bathtub" is still the most effective machine to fragment stones, the water bath is cumbersome, so bath-free versions of the ESWL machine were made. In these machines, instead of being lowered into a tub of water, the patient lies on a water cushion which allows transmission of the shock waves from the generator to the patient. ESWL can be used for kidney or ureteral stones, although the results are better for kidney stones. The operation usually lasts 1 hour, and patients are generally treated with just intravenous sedation. Most patients are discharged home on the day of treatment with oral pain medication, and they can usually return to work one or two days after ESWL.

Once the stone is fragmented, it is hoped that the small pieces will pass down the ureter on their own. If the stone is greater than 1 cm. in diameter, there is a risk that the stone fragments can bunch up and block the ureter as they pass (a condition known as steinstrasse). To avoid this complication, some people recommend cystoscopy and ureteral stent placement on the side of the stone before ESWL. The stent can usually be removed a few days after a successful ESWL. Some risks of ESWL include:

- Infection.
- Bleeding around the kidney (since the kidney moves up and down with breathing, shock waves sometimes hit normal kidney tissue instead of the stone).
- The need for transfusion.
- The need for open surgery to stop renal bleeding.
- Pain.
- Failure to fragment the stone.
- Residual stone fragments which might require a second ESWL.
- High blood pressure.
- Damage to adjacent structures (e.g., colon, spleen, and liver).
- Steinstrasse from multiple stone fragments obstructing the ureter.
- Anesthetic risk.

If steinstrasse occurs, it is usually treated with the placement of a percutaneous nephrostomy tube for drainage of the kidney which results in subsequent passage of the fragments in approximately 72 percent of cases. The only absolute contraindication to ESWL is pregnancy. Bleeding disorders need to be corrected before ESWL as before any surgical procedure. Since an electrical charge is used to generate the shock waves in most ESWL machines, a cardiology consultation is usually obtained before ESWL if the patient has a pacemaker.

OPEN SURGERY

Many years ago, kidney stones were managed by making an incision in the patient's flank and cutting open the kidney to remove the stone. Stones in the ureter were removed through incisions in the side or lower abdomen. Patients stayed in the hospital for about one week and were out of work for a few weeks until they recovered from surgery. Today, stones that cannot pass spontaneously and become lodged in the upper urinary tract requiring surgical treatment can usually be managed with ESWL, percutaneous nephrostolithotripsy, ureteroscopic techniques, or some combination of these procedures. Only about 1 to 4 percent of all stones still require open surgical removal.

LOCATION OF STONES

Kidney Stone

For symptomatic stones less than 2.5 cm. in diameter, ESWL with or without stent placement is the recommended procedure with an 88 to 92 percent success rate. Asymptomatic patients sometimes choose observation with follow-up KUBs in 6 to 12 months. If the stone increases in size or causes symptoms, definitive treatment is indicated. For stones greater than 2.5 cm. in diameter, studies show that multiple ESWL procedures are usually required to achieve a stone-free state, so in these patients, PNL is the initial treatment of choice. If stone fragments remain, ESWL or repeat PNL may be needed. Very large stones with multiple side branches, known as staghorn calculi, usually require treatment with PNL to remove the bulk of the stone followed by ESWL to fragment the hard-to-reach pieces. As stated prior, open surgical removal is rarely necessary with today's technology.

Ureteral Stone

Many ureteral stones will pass spontaneously. Any ureteral stone less than 5 mm. in diameter can be expected to pass spontaneously in about 80 to 98 percent of cases, while stones greater than 8 mm. have only a 20 percent chance of passing on their own. Therefore, observation for up to 4 weeks is an option for stones up to 8 mm. in diameter as long as the patient's pain is controlled and some dye from the IVP can be seen to get passed the stone. In stones that fail to pass, or for stones greater than 8 mm. in size, surgical options should be considered. The surgical treatment of choice for upper ureteral stones is ESWL with or without stent placement. It has an excellent success rate and is minimally invasive. Stones that are not responsive to ESWL may require lithotripsy via a ureteroscope, but the need for this is rare. The need for open surgery to treat these stones is even rarer now.

For stones in the middle part of the ureter, ESWL has a success rate of about 80 percent, while the success rate for the treatment of these stones with ureteroscopic techniques approaches 60 to 70 percent. Although the success rates are similar, ESWL is less invasive, and it is, therefore, the procedure of choice to manage mid-ureteral stones as well. If ESWL fails, ureteroscopic techniques can then be attempted. Open surgery may be appropriate as a salvage procedure or in certain unusual circumstances.

Distal ureteral stones have a greater than 90 percent chance of being successfully removed with ureteroscopy. ESWL is less invasive than ureteroscopy, but it has a slightly lower success rate than ureteroscopy in the treatment of distal ureteral stones and may require multiple treatments for adequate fragmentation. Therefore, in lower ureteral stones that either fail to pass spontaneously or are significantly symptomatic, ureteroscopic removal with or without lithotripsy is usually recommended first. However, ESWL is an acceptable treatment option. Again, the need for open surgery is rare, and although it should not be considered first line treatment, open surgery may be appropriate as a salvage procedure or in nonstandard situations.

LIFE AFTER A STONE

Once a stone passes or is removed, it is sent to the laboratory to determine its chemical composition. This is important since knowledge of the type of stone can help in making recommendations for the prevention of future stones. Measures to prevent future stones are crucial since after passing one stone, a person has a 15 percent chance of getting another stone within one year and a 50 percent chance of getting another stone within 4 to 5 years.

After the passage of one stone, most physicians usually recommend increased fluid intake and various dietary modifications; however, after a second stone, an extensive evaluation including a 24 hour urine collection to search for excessive urinary excretion of certain stone constituents is usually undertaken.

The single-most important modification that can be recommended for all stone-forming patients is a high fluid intake. Patients are recommended to drink one gallon of fluid per day, half of which is water or enough fluid to achieve greater than 2.5 liters of urine output per day. Patients who live in hot climates or whose job entails physical exertion are recommended to drink even more than this, since more fluid is lost as sweat rather than being excreted in the urine predisposing to lower urine volumes and supersaturation. An attempt should be made to keep the intake of fluid as consistent throughout the day and night as possible.

Patients are usually encouraged to eliminate dietary excesses, especially protein or foods rich in oxalate or calcium. Moderate salt restriction has also been shown to decrease the risk of calcium stone formation. Also, in the 20 percent of calcium stone patients who have elevated levels of uric acid in their urine, allopurinol (a drug used in the treatment of gout) has been recommended to decrease the risk of stones. Diuretics such as hydro-chlorothiazide can decrease the excretion of calcium into the urine and are sometimes used in calcium stone formers to try to prevent further stones.

The prevention of uric acid stones consists of increased fluid intake to keep urine volumes greater than 2 liters per day, limiting dietary protein to less than 90 grams per day, and alkalinizing the urine to a pH between 6.5 and 7.0 with either sodium bicarbonate or potassium citrate. Allopurinol may also decrease the production of uric acid by the body and thus, decrease the risk of uric acid stone formation.

Prevention of cystine stones also consists of high fluid intake and urinary alkalinization (to a pH greater than 7.5). A low sodium diet has also been suggested to decrease the risk of cystine stone formation. In resistant cases, there are various drugs that can be used to improve the solubility of cystine in the urine.

The prevention of infection stones requires the maintenance of sterile urine with long-term suppressive antibiotics, high urine volumes, and limiting dietary phosphate intake. Adherence to these preventive measures is crucial since the recurrence rate of infection stones is approximately 30 percent by six years after treatment.

BLADDER STONES

Bladder stones sometimes originate as kidney stones that pass into the bladder; however, they usually tend to form in the bladder in men with an enlarged prostate or with neurologic problems that prevent complete bladder emptying. In patients whose prostatic enlargement prevents complete bladder emptying, retained urine can become concentrated and/or infected, predisposing them to the formation of bladder stones. These patients usually have some degree of voiding symptoms, such as decreased force of stream, hesitancy, straining to void, or frequent urination. Patients with bladder stones may also have hematuria or sudden pain associated with an interrupted urine stream as the stone obstructs the bladder outlet like a ball valve. The diagnosis of a bladder stone is usually confirmed with either x-rays or cystoscopy. Bladder stones can usually be treated with cystoscopic removal with or without lithotripsy (e.g., electrohydraulic, laser, or ultrasonic). Open stone removal is occasionally necessary.

In summary, while most stones will pass spontaneously, sometimes people will need surgery to treat them. Although some of the newer treatment methods may be much nicer than open surgery, the best solution is to avoid getting a stone. For this reason, remember this "fluid ounce of prevention": drink water, water, and more water!

References

1. Gillenwater JY, Grayhack JT, Howards SS, and Duckett JW (eds.): *Adult and Pediatric Urology*, 3rd ed. St. Louis: Mosby, 1996.
2. Macfarlane MT: *Urology for the House Officer*, 2nd ed. Baltimore: Williams and Wilkins, 1995.
3. Segura JW, Preminger GM, Assimos DG, Dretler SP, Kahn RI, Lingeman JE, and Macaluso JN: "Ureteral Stones Clinical Guidelines Panel Summary Report on the Management of Ureteral Calculi." *J Urol* 1997, 158(5):1915-1921.

CHAPTER 20

BENIGN PROSTATIC HYPERPLASIA

As discussed in Chapter 16, the prostate is an accessory sex gland that sits just below the bladder and through which passes the urethra (see Figure 20-1). Its secretions aid in the transport of sperm during ejaculation, and also help to liquefy the semen. However, the prostate is most known for the problems it can cause. Prostatitis was discussed in Chapter 16, and prostate cancer is addressed in Chapter 21. This chapter reviews the evaluation and management of benign prostatic hyperplasia.

At birth, the prostate is about the size of a pea. As men age, the prostate undergoes benign enlargement, which has been termed benign prostatic hyperplasia (BPH). As the prostate enlarges, it can constrict the urethra and may cause problems with urination.

BPH is the most common non-cancerous form of cell growth in men, accounting for over 1.7 million office visits and nearly 400,000 surgical procedures each year in the United States. Based on autopsy studies, pathologic evidence of BPH can be found in up to 30 percent of men at age 50, and in approximately 80 percent of men at age 80. It has been estimated that up to 30 percent of men between 50 and 80 years of age will undergo some form of treatment for BPH. It should be stressed that BPH is a benign condition (i.e., non-cancerous), and it has no relation to prostate cancer except that both conditions tend to occur in older patients.

The cause of BPH is still unclear but its relationship to aging is well documented. It is believed that over time, hormonal imbalances between androgens (male hormones) and estrogens (female hormones) may stimulate prostatic growth. Some theories involve prostatic growth factors which are proteins that may be produced in response to hormonal factors. These growth factors may stimulate prostatic enlargement. Some studies suggest that BPH results from a decrease in the rate of cell death rather than an increase in the rate of cell proliferation.

There are some patients who have symptoms of BPH without having enlarged prostates. In these cases, it is believed that the muscles in and around the prostate contract to compress the prostatic tissue which in turn constricts the urethra resulting in the classic symptoms of bladder outlet obstruction. A family history of BPH may increase a man's chances of developing this condition.

Although BPH is rarely life-threatening, as the prostate enlarges, it can progressively constrict the urethra, causing bladder outlet obstruction that results in a variety of symptoms which urologists have termed prostatism:

- Decreased force and caliber of urinary stream.
- Hesitancy (having to wait in front of the toilet until enough pressure can be generated to begin urination).
- Having to strain to begin urination.
- Interruption of urinary stream (urine flow starts and stops a number of times during urination).
- Post-void dribbling (dribbling at the end of urination).
- Urgency (difficulty holding one's urine or feeling of need to urinate immediately).
- Nocturia (need to get up at night to urinate).
- Feeling of incomplete emptying.
- Hematuria (from strain on blood vessels in the bladder and prostate).
- Urinary retention (inability to void).

As BPH develops and constricts the flow of urine in the urethra, increasing bladder outlet resistance, the bladder responds by increasing its muscle tone, just like what happens when someone lifts weights. In the early stages, the hypertrophied bladder becomes irritable, or sensitive --that is, even small amounts of urine in the bladder may trigger the urge to urinate. The symptoms in this "irritable" phase may involve only decreased force of stream and nocturia. As the obstruction progresses, the bladder takes time to generate increased pressures to overcome the outlet resistance, so symptoms of hesitancy, straining to void, interrupted stream, and post-void dribbling may be noted. When outlet obstruction becomes severe, the bladder may not be able to force all the urine by the blockage, resulting in some urine remaining in the bladder after each voiding episode (i.e., residual urine). In these later stages, patients typically complain of feelings of incomplete emptying, recurrent urinary tract infections (due to retained urine), bladder stones (also due to retained urine), and urinary retention. Of note, the symptoms of BPH may be especially noticeable after drinking alcoholic beverages, taking decongestants, or being in cold weather.

Other conditions that can cause voiding problems similar to those that may be seen in BPH include: 1) bladder cancer; 2) urinary tract infections (e.g., prostatitis); 3) stones; 4) prostate cancer; 5) urethral strictures (narrowing of the urethra from scar tissue); and 6) side effects of certain medications. Since many different conditions can cause similar voiding dysfunction, it is recommended that any man with problems urinating consult a physician for further evaluation.

As in any medical problem, the keys to an accurate diagnosis are a detailed history, a thorough physical examination, and certain laboratory tests and special studies.

HISTORY

The history is aimed at a search for symptoms of prostatism. In addition, many physicians now have the patient fill out a form called the AUA Symptom Questionnaire to develop a symptom score to try to estimate the severity of the patient's voiding symptoms and how much they bother the patient (see Table 20-1). This questionnaire helps physicians grade the degree of the patient's symptoms into mild (total score of 0 to 7), moderate (total score of 8 to 19), and severe (total 20 to 35). Since the treatment of BPH often depends on how much patients are bothered by their symptoms, the AUA Symptom Questionnaire sometimes plays an important part in helping to decide on treatment options.

A significant number of patients with BPH-induced outlet obstruction present with acute urinary retention. Sudden distention of the bladder is usually felt as severe pain in the lower abdomen just above the penis and a persistent urge to void. This situation may be precipitated by ingestion of

Table 20-1: AUA Symptom Questionnaire for Benign Prostatic Hyperplasia (Circle one number each line)						
Symptom	Not at all	Less than 1 time in 5	Less than half the time	About half the time	More than half the time	Almost always
Over the past month, how often have you had a sensation of not emptying your bladder after you finished urinating?	0	1	2	3	4	5 or more
Over the past month, how often have you had to urinate again less than two hours after you finished urinating?	0	1	2	3	4	5 or more
Over the past month, how often have you found that you stopped and started again several times when you urinated?	0	1	2	3	4	5 or more
Over the past month, how often have you found it difficult to postpone urination?	0	1	2	3	4	5 or more
Over the past month, how often have you had a weak urinary stream?	0	1	2	3	4	5 or more
Over the past month, how often have you had to push or strain to begin urination?	0	1	2	3	4	5 or more
Over the past month, how many times did you most typically get up to urinate from the time you went to bed at night until the time you got up in the morning?	0	1	2	3	4	5 or more
Add up the sum of all the answers circled:	Total score: 0-7 = mild symptoms 8-19 = moderate symptoms 20-35 = severe symptoms					

From: Reprinted with the permission of the American Urologic Association.

certain decongestants or tranquilizers, a delay in voiding, or with overdistention of the bladder as occurs with ingestion of alcohol or diuretics.

Recurrent urinary tract infections may suggest bladder outlet obstruction with poor bladder emptying. Patients with BPH can also present with hematuria, either gross or microscopic.

A thorough history, including medications, past medical and past surgical history, is also necessary, since it may uncover other conditions that can mimic the symptoms of BPH. Also, the patient's overall medical condition often plays a role in determining the final treatment plan.

PHYSICAL EXAMINATION

On physical exam, a distended bladder may be palpated in the patient in urinary retention. The digital rectal examination (DRE) is used to examine the prostate. During the DRE, the physician inserts a gloved, lubricated finger a few inches into the patient's rectum and evaluates the prostate for size, nodularity (which may suggest prostate cancer), or tenderness (which may suggest prostatitis). If any suspicious areas are found on DRE, a prostate biopsy may be recommended for further evaluation (see Chapter 21). Not everyone with an enlarged prostate on DRE has difficulty voiding, and there are many patients with small prostates on DRE who have significant outlet obstructive symptoms.

LABORATORY STUDIES

A *urinalysis* is usually performed to detect hematuria, infection, or other conditions that can cause symptoms similar to those seen with BPH.

A *serum creatinine* is a blood test used to evaluate the patient's kidney function. As renal function deteriorates, the serum creatinine level increases. Approximately 13 percent of patients with BPH will develop some degree of kidney problems.

Prostate specific antigen (PSA) is a protein made almost exclusively by the prostate to help liquefy the semen. It can be elevated in men with enlarged prostate glands, prostatitis, or prostate cancer, and it is the standard screening test for prostate cancer. A yearly DRE and PSA test are generally recommended for men aged 50 and older, and for men aged 40 and over who are at high risk for prostate cancer (positive family history, or those of African descent). Up to 50 percent of men with BPH experience a moderate rise in PSA, while in 10 percent of patients with BPH, the PSA may be higher than 10 ng/ml. In patients with an elevated PSA level, a prostate biopsy may be recommended to search for the presence of prostate cancer. PSA is discussed in more detail in Chapter 21.

SPECIAL STUDIES

In most patients, additional tests are usually recommended only to help make decisions regarding treatment options or to rule out other causes of certain symptoms.

A *uroflow test* tries to evaluate the velocity of urine flow. When the patient's bladder is full, he is asked to urinate into a funnel-like device that measures the flow of urine in milliliters per second and the volume of urine excreted in milliliters. The theory is that a healthy person should be able to void a relatively large amount of urine in a short time; whereas less urine is able to flow through the obstructed area per unit of time. For example, a peak flow of greater than 18 ml/sec is usually normal. A peak flow of 10 to 15 ml/sec may indicate moderate BPH, and a peak flow rate of less than 10 ml/sec may be a sign of severe BPH. The problem is that a weak bladder, as seen in some patients with neurologic disorders, may also not be able to generate enough pressure to give rise to a normal flow rate and, thus, the peak flow will be low. Therefore, uroflow tests can't really differentiate between bladder outlet obstruction and a weak bladder.

A *post-void residual test* (PVR) measures the amount of urine remaining in the bladder after urination. This test can be performed by passing a small catheter up the urethra and into the bladder (which is the most accurate method but slightly uncomfortable) or by using ultrasound to measure the size of the bladder to help estimate the amount of residual urine. A "normal" PVR value has not yet been determined; however, it has been suggested that a PVR greater than 60 to 100 ml. is excessive, indicating either significant outlet obstruction or a weak bladder, and requires further evaluation.

A pressure-flow study uses a small catheter passed up the urethra into the bladder to measure bladder pressures during the performance of a uroflow test. Low bladder pressures in the presence of high flow rates indicate normal function. High bladder pressures with low flow rates indicates outlet obstruction due to BPH or urethral stricture. Low bladder pressures with low flow rates suggest a weak bladder. Not all urologists have access to machines that can perform these studies.

As discussed earlier, in cystoscopy, the urethra is filled with an anesthetic jelly and a thin telescope is passed up the urethra into the bladder. The size of the prostate and the degree of bladder outlet obstruction can be determined. Other problems associated with BPH, such as bladder stones, may also be diagnosed. Although this procedure doesn't really help urologists make recommendations for treatment early on, if it is determined that the patient with BPH needs surgical management, then cystoscopy in the office may be helpful in evaluating the size of the prostate which is an important factor in deciding on the type of surgery to recommend. The risks of office cystoscopy are minimal, and include infection, bleeding, discomfort (especially when passing through the prostatic urethra), urethral stricture, and urinary retention.

In the past, evaluation of the upper urinary tract (the kidneys and ureters) by IVP or ultrasound was commonplace in patients with symptomatic BPH. Now, however, these studies are no longer recommended in patients with BPH unless other problems that warrant radiographic evaluation are present (e.g., hematuria, recurrent urinary tract infections, or history of kidney stones).

As stated earlier, not all voiding problems are due to BPH. Therefore, men who have voiding symptoms similar to those described in this chapter are advised to see their doctor for further evaluation. If it is determined that the patient does have BPH, there are a variety of treatment options available, but it must be stressed that an enlarged prostate alone is not reason enough to undergo treatment. Many men live with BPH for years without it affecting the quality of their lives.

The currently accepted criteria for intervention to relieve bladder neck obstruction due to BPH include:

- Urinary retention (the risk of retention in patients with BPH is 5 to 20 percent, and the risk of recurrent episodes of retention after draining the bladder is 70 percent).

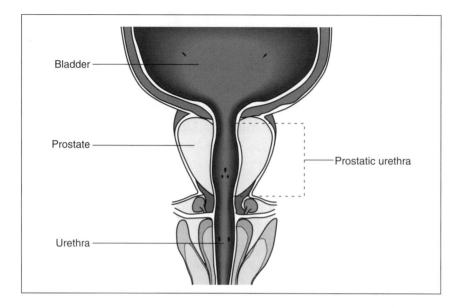

Figure 20-1: Schematic drawing of the lower urinary tract.

- Hydronephrosis (ureteral dilation from the back-up of retained urine due to prostatic obstruction).

- Recurrent urinary tract infection (due to residual urine).

- Bladder stone (due to residual urine).

- Gross hematuria (rare, but when evaluation rules out other sources, treatment is indicated for multiple episodes, especially when associated with clots or significant blood loss).

- Obstructive voiding symptoms that significantly interfere with the patient's quality of life (this is the most common indication for the treatment of BPH today).

TREATMENT

The primary goal of treatment for BPH is to decrease the patient's symptoms, presumably by improving urinary flow. The patient's perception of the severity of his condition, the presence of complications from BPH (e.g., urinary tract infections or bladder stones), and consultation with a urologist usually determine what treatment options are pursued. The various treatment options for BPH are usually divided into four major categories: 1) watchful waiting; 2) drug therapy; 3) major surgery; and 4) minimally invasive procedures.

WATCHFUL WAITING

In studies of patients with BPH who had their symptoms followed over time, about one-third had improvement in their symptoms, one-third got worse, and one-third stayed the same. Therefore, in patients with BPH but mild symptoms (for example, an AUA symptom score of 7 or below) or in patients with moderate symptoms (AUA score 8 to 19) who aren't too bothered by their condition, watchful waiting is a viable option. These patients are monitored every 6 to 12 months by a reassessment of their symptoms (usually by having them fill out another AUA symptom questionnaire), a DRE, and a PSA level. If their symptoms worsen, other treatment options can be pursued. If watchful waiting is chosen, certain lifestyle changes may help to relieve or avoid symptoms. For example, avoiding alcohol, coffee, or other fluids after dinner may help decrease nocturia. These patients are also advised to avoid decongestants, since such medications can prevent the muscles in the prostate and bladder neck area from relaxing and, thus, may increase bladder outlet obstructive symptoms. Antihistamines can also slow urine flow in men with BPH.

Patients with severe symptoms of BPH (AUA score 20 to 35) aren't good candidates for watchful waiting, and most of these patients are so bothered by their condition that they usually opt to do something to improve their symptoms.

DRUG THERAPY

The most effective treatments for BPH are usually the most invasive and carry the greatest risk of complications. In an attempt to avoid the complications which can be associated with surgery, other treatment options have been, and continue to be, developed. For example, certain drugs that improve voiding symptoms in patients with BPH have been discovered.

There are two types of drugs used to treat BPH. The first are 5-alpha reductase inhibitors, which shrink the prostate. The other type of drugs used to treat BPH are alpha-blockers, which relax the muscles in and around the prostate. It is now believed that alpha blockers are more likely to reduce the symptoms of BPH, irregardless of the size of the prostate, while 5-alpha reductase inhibitors may only help men with significantly enlarged prostates.

Unfortunately, sometimes these medications may take weeks to months to achieve an effect, so drug therapy may not be an acceptable choice for patients with urinary retention, recurrent urinary tract infections, high residual urine volumes, or bladder stones. Another problem is that the medications need to be taken for life, since once they are discontinued the symptoms of BPH invariably return.

5-alpha Reductase Inhibitors

Castration produces a marked decrease in the size of the prostate in the dog. Although it is a rather extreme option for a little problem with urination, this finding focused attention on the hormonal treatment of BPH. Finasteride (trade name Proscar) blocks the action of the enzyme 5-alpha reductase, which converts the male hormone testosterone into the more powerful hormone dihydrotestosterone (DHT). Inhibition of this enzyme causes the prostate to shrink, and may decrease the degree of urinary obstruction. This drug has been shown to reduce prostatic size by 30 percent in two-thirds of patients who take it. However, it can take up to three to six months to notice a change in symptoms, if there are any changes at all.

Proscar is usually prescribed in a dose of 5 mg. once-a-day, and it has few side effects, the most common of which include impotence (5 percent) and decreased sex drive (3 to 4 percent). Its average cost per year is between $700 and $1400. Recently, Proscar was reported to be no better than a placebo in improving the symptoms of BPH; however, in this study, the majority of patients had only normal or moderately enlarged prostate glands. It is now suggested that Proscar may be helpful for men with symptomatic BPH who are found to have very large prostates. In this group of patients, decreasing the size of the prostate may relieve their obstructive voiding symptoms.

It is important to note that Proscar reduces prostate specific antigen (PSA) levels, which can obscure screening test results for prostate cancer if this side effect is not considered. Therefore, in patients who have been on Proscar for longer than three months, the PSA result should be doubled to calculate their actual PSA level.

It has been suggested that Proscar may have favorable results in the treatment of recurrent bleeding due to BPH. In addition, studies are currently in progress to evaluate whether Proscar is effective in preventing prostate cancer. Results of this study will not be available for several years. Proscar is also being evaluated as a possible treatment for male-pattern baldness, but again, it may take several years to complete these studies.

Alpha Blockers

These drugs relax the smooth muscles in and around the prostate, decreasing the amount of pressure on the urethra, which may increase urinary flow and improve voiding symptoms. Alpha blockers are taken once-a-day, usually at bedtime, and symptomatic improvement tends to occur within four to six weeks. If symptoms don't improve within one to two months, other types of treatment should be considered.

Doxazosin (trade name Cardura) and terazosin (trade name Hytrin) are the alpha blockers commonly used in the treatment of BPH. Another alpha blocker, known as tamsulosin (trade name Flomax), has recently been approved by the FDA for patients with symptomatic BPH. Initial results have shown Flomax to be similar to the other alpha blockers in effectiveness, but because it is believed to work more specifically on prostatic smooth muscle, it may have fewer side effects than Cardura or Hytrin.

Alpha blockers may cause a lowering of blood pressure if the patient stands up rapidly (orthostatic hypotension), resulting in dizziness or light-headedness (2 to 5 percent). This risk can be reduced by taking the medication at bedtime. These drugs can also cause nasal congestion, drowsiness or headache (10 to 15 percent), retrograde ejaculation (4 to 11 percent), and impotence (2 percent). Their average cost per year is between $700 and $1400.

151

Phytotherapeutic Agents

Phytotherapy is defined as the use of plants or plant extracts for medical purposes, and has been described since ancient times. These agents are popular because patients with chronic conditions are often tempted to try alternative treatments. Most of the phytotherapeutic agents commonly used today are plant extracts rather than the plant itself.

The most widely used phytotherapeutic agent for BPH is the extract of the saw palmetto berry (saw palmetto is a dwarf palm tree native to the West Indies and southeastern United States). It has been suggested that saw palmetto may block the production of dihydrotestosterone, but clinical studies in humans have not yielded any definitive data on its mechanism of action. Furthermore, although some small studies have suggested that saw palmetto is helpful in improving the symptoms of BPH, the most definitive studies have shown no significant difference between saw palmetto and placebo.

Other agents that have been used in an attempt to improve symptomatic BPH include: cernilton (pollen extract), Pygeum africanum (African plum) or its extract tadenan, and urtica or bazoton (extracts of the plant *Radix urticae*). Prosata is the trade name of a medication that can be purchased without a prescription, and is basically a mixture of multiple plant extracts, including *Pygeum africanum* and *Urtica dioica*. These items are often found listed in the "ingredients" section on the labels of some over-the-counter "prostate" medications. Since they are considered alternative medicines, most doctors don't prescribe them. But they are usually advertised in men's magazines or are found in health food stores.

One problem in evaluating these and any treatment for BPH is the placebo effect. A placebo is a harmless substance given as medicine, like a sugar pill. Studies have shown that approximately 30 to 40 percent of patients with symptomatic BPH will report improvement in their symptoms when unknowingly treated with a placebo. Therefore, when evaluating any new treatment for BPH, this placebo effect must be taken into account (preferably by including a "placebo group" in the study). It should also be remembered that it is dangerous to assume that "natural" substances have no side effects and are completely safe.

Evidence for the efficacy of phytotherapeutic agents in the treatment of BPH is inconclusive, and currently, these agents are believed to be no more than an expensive form of placebo. So, until scientific studies determine the actual benefits, proper dosages, and side effects of non-regulated herbal products, the patient is at risk for ineffective or even harmful treatments.

MAJOR SURGERY

Transurethral resection of the prostate (TURP) and open prostatectomy are two surgical procedures that can be used to treat prostatism.

Transurethral Resection of the Prostate (TURP)

This procedure, commonly called the "roto-rooter job," is the most common operation for the treatment of BPH, with approximately 250,000 cases performed in the United States each year. During a TURP, the patient is under general or spinal anesthesia and the urologist passes a cystoscope up the urethra into the bladder. Then, using an electrified wire loop, obstructing prostatic tissue is cut away from the urethra. If the prostate were a lemon, the pulp is scraped out, leaving the peel behind for urine to flow through. The operation usually lasts about 30 to 60 minutes, but depends on the size of the prostate gland. If present, bladder stones can sometimes be fragmented with a lithotriptor passed up through the cystoscope and subsequently removed (see Chapter 19), thus avoiding open surgery. At the end of the operation, a catheter is placed into the bladder via the urethra, and continuous bladder irrigation is used for a few hours to keep the catheter patent until the bleeding stops. The catheter is usually removed on the second post-operative day. However, when a large amount of tissue is resected (e.g., greater than 30 grams), the catheter may be left in place for a few days longer and subsequently be removed in the office. With the push towards shorter hospital stays, many patients are now being discharged home on the day of surgery, but some patients who require longer observation are discharged home on the first or second post-operative day. Men can usually return to work in about one week, but they are advised to avoid aspirin products, strenuous activity, and heavy lifting for two to four weeks to avoid post-operative bleeding.

The best predictor of a successful outcome after a TURP is how much bother the patient is experiencing from his BPH symptoms. TURP usually provides immediate and significant improvement in symptoms, flow rates, and residual urine, with 75 to 96 percent of patients reporting improvement post-operatively. In comparison, other less invasive treatment options have been shown to result in significantly less degrees of symptom improvement than TURP. However, TURP is an invasive procedure and, as such, not without risk (overall complication rate approximately 16 percent).

There are many potential complications of TURP. These may include:

1. Failure to void (6 percent), which is more common in patients who had urinary retention pre-operatively.

2. Bleeding: Blood tinged urine can occur for a few days after the procedure. Bleeding significant enough to require transfusion during surgery (2.5 percent) or after surgery (3.9 percent) is usually associated with large glands (over 60 grams) or prolonged catheterization to treat urinary retention before TURP. Occasionally, a scab may come loose, causing a sudden episode of gross hematuria. This bleeding usually resolves with drinking plenty of fluids, avoiding strenuous activity, and avoiding aspirin products.

3. Dysuria: Burning or discomfort on urination usually resolves after a few days but can persist for weeks until the raw areas in the prostatic urethra heal.

4. Epididymitis (0.2 to 6 percent).

5. Retrograde ejaculation (80 to 90 percent): This condition may occur because the muscles at the bladder neck (i.e., where the bladder meets the prostate) are resected during TURP. Once these muscles are resected, the bladder neck can no longer close off during ejaculation so some semen leaks into the bladder instead of being forced out the penis (see Chapter 7).

6. Urethral stricture (2.7 to 20 percent), which is scar tissue in the urethra that can occur from 3 weeks to a few months after TURP and may result in the recurrence of symptoms of BPH.

7. Bladder neck contracture (2 percent) which is scar tissue that closes off the site where the bladder meets the urethra. The risk of this problem is higher with small glands (i.e., less than 30 grams).

8. TURP syndrome (2 percent) which occurs as a result of excessive absorption of the fluid used for irrigation during this surgery. It can result in high blood pressure, visual changes, and even seizures if severe enough. The risk of TURP syndrome is higher with longer resection times; therefore, it is recommended that TURP not take longer than 1 to 1.5 hours. Larger glands that might require longer than one and a half hours to resect are better handled with open surgery to avoid this problem.

9. Bladder perforation (under 1 percent).

10. Incontinence: Leakage of urine associated with straining has been reported to occur in approximately 2 percent of patients, but total incontinence with leakage most or all of the time occurs in 0.1 to 0.7 percent of patients.

11. Impotence (3 to 13.7 percent): Various studies have reported impotence rates between 4 and 40 percent; however, how impotence was defined in each of the studies may have been responsible for the ranges reported. If the patient had difficulty having erections prior to surgery, there is a greater chance of impotence after TURP.

12. Persistent symptoms after surgery (10 percent): Approximately 70 percent of patients with irritative voiding symptoms (i.e., frequency, urgency, and nocturia) due to BPH can be expected to have relief of these symptoms within 6 months of TURP. The remaining 30 percent may respond to medications that relax the bladder muscles.

13. The need for repeat TURP has been reported in 3 to 17 percent of patients, but this is usually not necessary for at least seven to eight years after the original operation, if at all.

14. Headache after spinal anesthesia (2 percent).

15. Death (less than 1 percent).

The average cost of TURP is $4000 to $6000.

Open Prostatectomy

In this operation, the enlarged prostate is removed through an incision in the lower abdomen. It is usually performed under spinal or general anesthesia. The urologist gains access to the prostate by cutting through the bladder or by opening the prostatic capsule. Then, the prostatic tissue is scooped out with the surgeon's finger. Again, if the prostate were a grapefruit, the surgeon scoops out the pulp and leaves the peel. During this operation, other problems that can result from BPH can be treated as well (e.g., bladder stones can be removed). The operation usually takes about 1.5 to 2 hours. At the end of the procedure, a urethral catheter is placed for bladder irrigation and urinary drainage. The catheter is usually removed in seven to ten days. Most patients are discharged home with antibiotics and pain medication between five and seven days after the surgery, and return to the office to have their catheters removed. Patients are advised not to drive for a few days after discharge, and to avoid aspirin products, strenuous activity, and heavy lifting for four weeks after their surgery.

It should be noted that the open surgery to treat BPH is different than the open surgery used to treat prostate cancer. In treating prostate cancer, the entire prostate (capsule and all prostatic tissue) is removed, while in treating BPH only the obstructing prostatic tissue is scooped out, leaving some prostatic tissue behind to avoid the greater risk of complications associated with prostate cancer surgery.

Open prostatectomy is more invasive, requires a longer hospital stay, and carries a higher risk of complications than TURP. The majority of urologists today prefer TURP over open prostatectomy, except in cases in which the prostate is so large that it would take too long to adequately remove all of the obstructing tissue using TURP (i.e., glands larger than 80 to 100 grams). Therefore, only about 2 to 3 percent of patients with BPH are now treated with open prostatectomy. This procedure does, however, provide excellent relief of outlet obstructive symptoms, with a 94 to 100 percent reported success rate.

Since open prostatectomy is the most invasive treatment option for BPH, it is also associated with the greatest risk of complications, with an overall complication rate of 21 percent.

Some complications associated with this operation include:

1. Infection (3 to 10 percent).
2. Bleeding significant enough to require transfusion (30 percent).
3. Dysuria (similar to TURP).
4. Retrograde ejaculation (85 to 95 percent).
5. Bladder neck contracture (2 to 14 percent).
6. Incontinence (1 percent).
7. Impotence (7 to 10 percent).
8. Need for additional treatment for BPH within 8 years after surgery (10 percent).
9. Death (2 percent).

The average cost of open prostatectomy is $10,000 to $15,000.

MINIMALLY INVASIVE PROCEDURES

The previously mentioned complication data should not detract from the fact that approximately 90 percent of all men subjected to some form of prostatectomy to treat BPH benefit from the procedure. However, the desire to minimize morbidity and mortality associated with the management of BPH has led to the search for less invasive procedures.

Most minimally invasive therapies use heat to destroy prostatic tissue. Heat destruction can be achieved by high-frequency current, laser beams, microwaves, radio frequency (RF) current, or ultrasonic heating. Two other minimally invasive procedures that will be discussed in this section are balloon dilation and stents, both of which involve the mechanical separation or spreading of prostate tissue to try to relieve outlet obstructive symptoms.

Transurethral Incision of the Prostate

Cutting a ring in two places allows you to open up and enlarge the ring. Some patients with prostatism don't have enlarged prostates, and in these patients it is believed that the muscles in the bladder neck and prostatic capsule are so tense that they constrict the urethra, resulting in their obstructive symptoms. It is suggested that cutting through the bladder neck muscles and through the prostatic tissue to the prostatic capsule in two areas will open up the prostatic urethra and improve these patient's voiding symptoms. This procedure is called transurethral incision of the prostate (TUIP).

Although it has been carried out under local anesthesia, TUIP is usually performed under spinal or general anesthesia. Once adequate anesthesia is administered, a cystoscope, similar to that used for TURP, is passed up the urethra into the bladder and, using a type of knife (instead of the wire loop used for TURP), cuts are made in the bladder neck and through the entire length of the prostate down to the outermost layer of the prostate, the prostatic capsule. These cuts are usually made at the five and seven o'clock positions, and the operation usually takes 15 to 30 minutes. At the end of the procedure, a catheter is placed up the urethra for bladder irrigation and urinary drainage. The patient is usually discharged home on the day of surgery or the following morning, with the catheter hooked up to a drainage bag that wraps around the patient's leg. The catheter is removed in the office when the patient's urine is clear, which is usually 24 to 48 hours post-operatively.

Most studies have reported excellent success rates for TUIP, with a greater than 80 to 90 percent chance of symptom improvement. Since no prostate tissue is usually removed with TUIP, it is not recommended for large prostates with a lot of obstructing tissue. Most urologists recommend this procedure for patients with prostatism unresponsive to medical therapy but whose prostate glands are small on evaluation (less than 20 to 30 grams). In this group of patients, success rates of TUIP are identical to those for TURP with significantly less morbidity and length of hospital stay.

Some of the reported complications of TUIP include:

1. Infection (2 to 5 percent).

2. Bleeding significant enough to require blood transfusion (2 percent).

3. Retrograde ejaculation (15 to 20 percent), so in younger patients who might want to preserve ejaculatory function, especially if they have small prostate glands, TUIP is recommended over TURP to relieve outlet obstructive symptoms.

4. Urethral stricture (10 percent).

5. Bladder neck contracture: This is almost non-existent after TUIP, while it is fairly common after TURP in patients with small glands (i.e., less than 20 to 30 grams).

6. Impotence (2 to 4 percent).

7. Incontinence (1 percent).

8. Need for additional surgery to treat symptoms of BPH within eight years after TUIP (20 percent).

9. Death (less than 1 percent).

The average cost of TUIP is $2000 to $4000.

Transurethral Electrovaporization of the Prostate

Transurethral electrovaporization of the prostate (TVP) uses high voltage, high frequency electrical currents to vaporize obstructing prostatic tissue. TVP is performed under spinal or general anesthesia. During this operation, a cystoscope is passed up the urethra into the bladder. A round ball through which current flows (instead of the cutting loop used in TURP) is rolled over the prostate tissue. This causes the tissue to vaporize and any blood to coagulate. The operation usually lasts 30 to 60 minutes, depending on the size of the gland. A catheter is placed at the end of the procedure, and it is removed when the urine is clear (before discharge or 24 to 48 hours after TVP). The patients are usually discharged home on the day of surgery, with or without a catheter.

One disadvantage of TVP is the lack of tissue for pathologic evaluation. However, if tissue is needed, a TURP loop can be used to obtain prostate tissue samples for study. On the other hand, one advantage of TVP is that since prostate tissue is vaporized instead of being removed, there is minimal bleeding associated with this procedure.

Early success rates for TVP are similar to those for TURP. TVP also appears to have a lower incidence of complications than TURP, but long-term studies are needed to determine the "staying power" of this procedure.

Laser Prostatectomy

Laser energy can be used to either vaporize prostate tissue or to coagulate the tissue and seal off blood vessels with subsequent necrosis and sloughing of obstructing tissue over time. The procedure is performed on an outpatient basis under spinal or general anesthesia, but it has been done using only intravenous sedation and local anesthesia. Laser energy is delivered via a laser fiber introduced through a cystoscope, and the operation usually takes about 20 minutes. Most men require a temporary catheter to drain the bladder for a few days after surgery.

One advantage of this procedure is that blood loss is minimal. The most frequent complication from laser surgery is the requirement for prolonged (one to six weeks) catheter drainage in patients with urinary retention. Early results have shown that dysuria and other irritative voiding symptoms are more severe after laser prostatectomy than after TURP, and it can take weeks to months for the dead prostatic tissue to slough off and for maximal improvement in symptoms to occur. The reoperation rates in the first year are 5 to 10 percent, but the need for a second operation (usually a TURP) is even greater in patients presenting in urinary retention. Incontinence after this procedure has not been reported.

Recently approved by the FDA, the *interstitial laser* is now being used to treat symptomatic BPH. This procedure is performed on an outpatient basis under spinal or general anesthesia. In it, a fiberoptic plastic probe is passed through the cystoscope and is inserted directly into the prostate. Then, laser energy is used to destroy the prostatic tissue that is causing obstruction to urine flow. The procedure usually takes 15 to 30 minutes, and most men require a temporary catheter to drain the bladder for two to five days, depending on the size of their prostate. Patients may experience some frequency and urgency for a few weeks; however, most patients have reported improvement in their symptoms by four to six weeks after the procedure. The interstitial laser has been reported to have promising results with minimal risk of complications. As with any new treatment modality, however, longer follow-up is needed to determine its role in the treatment of patients with BPH.

The average cost of interstitial laser treatment is $2000 to $4000.

Transurethral Microwave Thermotherapy (TUMT)

In this procedure, microwave energy is used to heat and destroy prostatic tissue. The first device approved by the FDA for microwave treatment is the Prostatron. TUMT is usually performed in a single session without anesthesia or with mild sedation and local anesthesia. A microwave antenna is inserted up through the urethra and positioned at the level of the prostate using ultrasound guidance. Microwave pulses then pass through the antenna to heat the prostate. The antenna is covered by a cooling tube to prevent burning and subsequent stricture of the urethra. The microwave energy levels and cooling system are both controlled by computer. The procedure takes about one hour, and the patients usually go home immediately afterward. Since inflammation results from the heating process, patients usually require a urinary catheter for three to four days until the swelling resolves. Of note, the fixed length of the urethral microwave antenna requires a minimum prostatic urethral length of 3.5 cm; therefore, patients with smaller prostates are not candidates for TUMT at the present time.

Early results have shown that, although objective improvement (e.g., flow rate) is less pronounced than after TURP, overall symptomatic improvement is similar (80 percent for TUMT vs. 90 percent for TURP in one study).

Complications of TUMT have been very rare. The most common problem is transient urinary retention requiring temporary catheter drainage (36 percent). Other risks of this procedure include:

1. Urethral stricture.
2. Dysuria, which usually resolves in two to three weeks.
3. Hematuria.
4. Need for further surgery due to persistent symptoms (30 to 60 percent so far).

TUMT does not appear to significantly affect sexual function or cause incontinence or retrograde ejaculation.

The early bottom line on TUMT is that it is a simple, office-based procedure that requires little or no anesthesia and has minimal morbidity. It is probably as effective as medical treatment for BPH, with symptomatic improvement exceeding objective improvement. Long-term studies are still needed. For now, it appears that most patients will fail TUMT between one and four years after treatment, and a majority of these patients will eventually require additional treatment for symptomatic BPH.

The average cost of TUMT is $8000 to $10,000.

Transurethral Needle Ablation of the Prostate

In this procedure, radiofrequency energy can be transmitted through tissue. When this energy is absorbed by the tissue, localized heating and tissue destruction occur. Transurethral needle ablation of the prostate (TUNA) has recently been approved by the FDA for the treatment of BPH. The operation is performed on an outpatient basis under sedation and local anesthesia, although a few patients have required general anesthesia due to discomfort.

The instrument used for TUNA is a cystoscopic rigid rod with two retractable needle antennae shaped like a "V" which can be extruded from the tip of the instrument for placement into prostatic tissue. The TUNA instrument is passed up the urethra to the level of the prostate under direct vision. The needles are then extended from the tip of the instrument and inserted into one side of the prostate (e.g., the left side at the two and four o'clock positions). Once adequate positioning is achieved, radiofrequency emission is started and continued for a five minute application. After this, the needles are withdrawn and reinserted into the other side of the prostate (i.e., the right side at the eight and ten o'clock positions), and another treatment is performed.

The operation usually takes about 30 minutes, and patients are sent home on the day of surgery. Since 35 to 40 percent of patients have required temporary catheter placement for urinary retention after TUNA, most patients are now sent home with a catheter for urinary drainage, and the catheter is removed in the office two to five days later. Like other thermal approaches, it usually takes a few weeks for voiding symptoms to improve.

Short-term results with TUNA have been encouraging, although significantly less impressive than TURP. Durability of symptomatic relief after this procedure appears to be lacking, with 40 to 50 percent of patients requiring additional treatment for recurrent symptoms by two years postoperative follow-up.

Complications of TUNA are rare, and include:

1. Bleeding.

2. Dysuria and other irritative voiding symptoms which can last for days to weeks.

3. Transient urinary retention.

4. Recurrent outlet obstructive symptoms.

The risk of impotence, retrograde ejaculation, incontinence, and urethral stricture is almost non-existent with this procedure.

The average cost of TUNA is $2000 to $4000.

Ultrasound Therapy

Ultrasonic waves can be focused on the prostate to rapidly heat the tissue and result in necrosis and subsequent sloughing of obstructing tissue. This procedure has been called high-intensity focused ultrasound (HIFU). Ultrasound can also be used to mechanically disrupt obstructive prostatic tissue which can then be removed with a suction device, a procedure known as transurethral ultrasonic aspiration of the prostate. Early reports are encouraging, but these are still experimental procedures which require longer follow-up to determine their true place in the management of BPH.

Balloon Dilation of the Prostate (BDP)

This procedure involves inserting a balloon into the urethra through a catheter. When the balloon is positioned at the level of the prostatic urethra, it is inflated to compress the obstructing prostatic tissue and widen the urethra at this level. Balloon inflation is maintained for 10 to 15 minutes, after which time the balloon is deflated and withdrawn. Early reports were encouraging, but most long-term studies have shown very little improvement in urinary symptoms with this technique. Most urologists have concluded that the chance of achieving a sustained improvement in voiding symptoms following BDP is not significant enough to justify this treatment for BPH. As a result, BDP is rarely offered today.

Prostatic Stents

The placement of a urethral catheter to drain the bladder in men with bladder outlet obstruction due to BPH is the simplest invasive treatment for this condition. Unfortunately, however, long-term indwelling catheters are uncomfortable and associated with many complications, especially urinary tract infections. Stents are hollow coils made of various metals that are placed via cystoscopy into the urethra at the level of the prostate and which spring open to expand the urethra in areas of narrowing. In essence, they are a form of completely internalized catheters.

Prostatic stent placement can be done on an outpatient basis under local or spinal anesthesia and usually takes about 15 minutes. Some stents are designed for temporary use, while others are meant to stay in place for indefinite periods of time.

Early results revealed that stents significantly increased urine flow, but between 8 and 37 percent of the stents needed to be removed later due to complications, such as dysuria, urinary tract infections, and persistent symptoms. This mode of treatment is still at the experimental stage, so little is known about long-term adverse effects. At the present time, it seems that there may be a place for permanent stents in the treatment of high-risk patients with limited life expectancy who can't tolerate other treatment options, and for temporary stents which could be placed after minimally invasive procedures to avoid temporary external catheters.

The average cost of prostatic stents is $2000 to $4000.

Benign prostatic hyperplasia is a common, almost unavoidable, problem in aging men. The number and variety of treatment options for symptomatic BPH continue to increase. For those men who have mild or tolerable symptoms, watchful waiting with a yearly DRE and PSA level is a viable option. When symptoms progress to become moderate or severe, a trial of medical therapy is usually recommended and may help some patients to avoid the need for more invasive treatments. For those patients who fail to respond to medical therapy, TURP has been the "gold standard" treatment for glands smaller than 70 to 80 grams, while open prostatectomy is usually recommended for patients with large prostates (greater than 80 to 100 grams). Symptomatic patients with small prostates (less than 30 grams) who are unresponsive to medical therapy may undergo transurethral incision of the prostate. The symptom outcome is equivalent to TURP, but patients experience much less morbidity. Transurethral electrovaporization of the prostate also seems to be an exciting and effective new modality. As for the other minimally invasive procedures, although they have fewer risks than TURP, they also tend to be less effective and less durable. Some patients are willing to sacrifice a little on efficacy to decrease the risk of complications, while others (usually those with more severe voiding symptoms) are not. Although TURP and open prostatectomy have proven themselves to be effective treatment options, more long-term studies are needed to determine which minimally invasive procedures will benefit which patients and which of these modalities will stand the test of time.

References

1. Gillenwater JY, Grayhack JY, Howards SS, and Duckett JW (eds.): *Adult and Pediatric Urology*, 3rd ed. St. Louis: Mosby, 1996.

2. Health Information Network, Inc.: *The Health Information Network: Benign Prostatic Hyperplasia (BPH): A Guide for Men.* HIN Inc.: San Ramon, CA, 1996.

3. Kabalin JN: "Invasive Therapies for Benign Prostatic Hyperplasia." *Monographs in Urology* 1997, 18(3):51-79.

4. Kahn SA and Narayan P: "Minimally Invasive Procedures for the Treatment of Symptomatic Benign Prostatic Hyperplasia." *Mediguide to Urology* 1997; 10(3):1-8.

5. Kapoor DA and Reddy PK: "Surgical Alternatives to TURP in the Management of BPH." *AUA Update Series* 1993; vol. 12, lesson 3.

6. Lepor H, et al: "The Efficacy of Terazosin, Finasteride, or Both in Benign Prostatic Hyperplasia." *New Engl J Med* 1996; 335(8):533-539.

7. Lowe FC and Ku JC: "Phytotherapy in Treatment of Benign Prostatic Hyperplasia: A Critical Review." *Urology* 1996; 48(1):12-20.

8. Macfarlane MT: *Urology for the House Officer*, 2nd ed. Baltimore: Williams and Wilkins, 1995.

9. Mebust WK: "BPH Patient Care Policies/Guidelines." *AUA Update Series* 1993; vol. 12, lesson 29.

10. Mebust WK: "Transurethral Prostatectomy." *AUA Update Series* 1994; vol. 13, lesson 18.

11. Oesterling JE and Moyad MA: *The ABC's of Prostate Cancer.* Lanham, MD: Madison Books, 1997.

12. Simm, Harvey (ed.): *Well-Connected: Benign Prostatic Hyperplasia.* Report # 71. New York: Nidus Information Services, Nov. 15, 1996.

13. Vaughan ED and Lepor H: "Medical Management of BPH: Part 1." *AUA Update Series* 1996; vol. 15, lesson 3.

CHAPTER 21

PROSTATE CANCER

To review, the prostate is an accessory sex gland located just below the bladder and through which passes the urethra (see Chapter 20). It is most famous, or should I say infamous, for the problems it can cause in life. Prostatitis and BPH have already been discussed, and in this chapter, the focus will be on prostate cancer.

There are many different cell types that make up the prostate and which can become cancerous. However, 95 percent of all prostate cancers are made up of glandular elements and are called adenocarcinomas. Adenocarcinoma of the prostate is what urologists are usually referring to when they talk about "prostate cancer." In fact, the remainder of this discussion will concern only adenocarcinoma of the prostate.

Prostate cancer is a very important health issue. It is the most common cancer in American males, other than superficial skin cancer, with an estimated 209,000 new cases diagnosed in 1997. It is the second most common cause of cancer deaths, behind lung cancer, with an estimated 41,800 deaths in 1997. Autopsy studies have shown that prostate cancer can be found in up to 30 percent of men 50 years of age and up to 70 to 80 percent of men at age 80. In fact, it is said that if a man lives long enough, he will eventually develop prostate cancer.

Many patients want to know how they got cancer. Although nobody really knows what causes prostate cancer, there are certain characteristics that increase a person's chances of being diagnosed with prostate cancer.

Some of these risk factors for prostate cancer include:

1. Increasing age.
2. Race: Blacks are twice as likely to develop prostate cancer than members of any other race in the world, while Asians, Hispanics, and Native American Indians have the lowest risk of developing prostate cancer.
3. High levels of testosterone.

167

4. Family history of prostate cancer: The average man's risk of getting prostate cancer is between 10 to 15 percent, but if one family member has had prostate cancer, the risk is double. If two family members have had prostate cancer, the risk is two to five times higher than in the general population. Of note, in people with a family history of prostate cancer, there is also an increased risk of developing it at an earlier age.

5. High fat diet: It is believed that a diet which is high in fat and low in fiber increases a person's chances of developing prostate cancer.

6. Decreased ultraviolet light exposure: It has been suggested that ultra-violet light from the sun has a protective effect against prostate cancer, therefore, decreased exposure to the sun may increase the risk of prostate cancer. This theory is supported by the observation that, in the United States, there is a higher rate of prostate cancer deaths in the North than in the South.

7. Vitamin D deficiency.

8. Chronic renal failure: The incidence of prostate cancer in these patients has been reported to be 1.8 times greater than in the general population.

Also, certain occupations (for example, those who work in water treatment, aircraft manufacturing, or with batteries or paint) and occupa-tional exposures (to chemicals such as metallic dust, cadmium exposure, lubricating oils, or pesticides) may be associated with a slight increased risk of prostate cancer. Recently, it has been suggested that men who have 22 or more alcoholic drinks per week increase their risk of getting prostate cancer.

Some factors that may *decrease* a person's risk of prostate cancer include:

1. Low-fat, high fiber diet.

2. Increased exposure to ultraviolet light.

3. Increased amounts of vitamin D (within the daily recommended allow-ance).

4. Lycopene, a pigment found in fresh tomatoes or tomato sauce (Mom, thanks for all those Sunday pasta dinners!).

5. Soy products.

6. Tea.

Factors believed to *not* have any effect on a person's risk for or against developing prostate cancer include:

1. Vasectomy: Recent studies have concluded that vasectomy does not increase one's risk of getting prostate cancer. In fact, the World Health Organization has stated that "any causal relationship between vasectomy and the risk of prostate cancer is unlikely." It has been suggested that since most vasectomies are performed by urologists, these patients are more likely to have their prostates checked regularly. More studies are being carried out to try to answer this question.

2. Smoking (but since it's responsible for so many other cancers, you should not smoke anyway).

3. Sexually transmitted diseases.

4. Frequency of sexual intercourse or number of sexual partners.

5. Benign prostatic hyperplasia (BPH).

6. Family history of other cancers.

DIAGNOSIS

Prostate cancer has been a disease of the elderly with approximately 75 percent of patients diagnosed between the ages of 60 and 85, and less than 2 percent of patients diagnosed under age 45. One principle that has been repeated throughout this book is that making a diagnosis of any disease process involves the history obtained from the patient, performing a physical examination, and various laboratory and special studies. The difficulty with prostate cancer is that, usually, this disease doesn't cause symptoms until it is in an advanced stage. While some people say, "If it ain't broke, don't fix it," others believe that we need to diagnose prostate cancer before it causes problems in order to find it at a curable stage and, hopefully, to save lives.

Screening

Screening is defined as a systematic program to detect a disease in a large population of asymptomatic people with the hope of reducing the death rate from this disease. In other words, you look for prostate cancer in men without symptoms in an attempt to find it at a curable stage. Early detection programs target populations considered at high risk for prostate cancer due to the presence of risk factors, such as family history, African-American heritage, or the other factors listed earlier.

The two tests that have been recommended to screen for prostate cancer have been a yearly digital rectal examination (DRE) and assessment of prostate specific antigen (PSA) level. It is assumed that early treatment initiated as a result of screening will be more effective than therapy undertaken at the usual time of diagnosis. This idea is good in theory, but to date, screening has not been conclusively proven to reduce the morbidity and mortality due to prostate cancer. In fact, opponents of screening for prostate cancer raise the possibility that prostate cancer may be discovered in patients who might never have developed symptoms from that cancer. Yet, a recent decline in prostate cancer death rates has been noted in the United States. These statistics suggest that screening, or early detection programs, may improve survival in men with prostate cancer. A National Cancer Institute (NCI) study is in progress to resolve the controversy over screening for this cancer, but it will take several years to be completed. In the meantime, most urologists feel that early detection of prostate cancer is beneficial.

The most efficient and cost-effective methods for the early detection of prostate cancer are the DRE and serum PSA level tests. It is recommended that men 50 years of age or older get a yearly DRE and PSA level by their physician. In those men at higher risk for prostate cancer (i.e., black men or those with a family history of prostate cancer), it is recommended that annual DRE and PSA level tests be started at age 40. If any questions arise with regard to the DRE or PSA level, the patient is usually referred to a urologist for further evaluation.

Another controversy revolves around when to cease annual DRE and PSA checks. However, once the patient's life expectancy becomes less than 10 years, the benefits of prostate cancer screening are minimal. For this reason, most physicians don't push annual prostate screening once the patient reaches 75 to 80 years of age, but the final decision of when to cease such examinations is between the patient and his physician.

History

As stated earlier, prostate cancer usually doesn't cause symptoms until it has progressed to an advanced stage; that is, until it has spread outside the prostate. In fact, patients often ask how they can have prostate cancer when they feel so good. However, sometimes prostate cancer can enlarge and constrict the urethra, causing all of the symptoms in the prostatism complex associated with BPH (see Chapter 20). The difference is that in patients with BPH, these symptoms tend to progress slowly over time, whereas in prostate cancer, these symptoms tend to get worse at a more rapid rate. Hematuria and hematospermia can also be signs of prostate cancer. When prostate cancer spreads outside the gland, patients may present with bone pain, weight loss, low blood counts, shortness of breathe, swelling in the legs from retained fluid, lower extremity weakness or paralysis from involvement of the spinal cord by their cancer, and urinary retention.

Physical Examination

The digital rectal examination (DRE) is the simplest and most common preliminary test for prostate cancer. During this procedure, the patient removes or drops his pants and is positioned in one of three ways: 1) bent over from the hips (sometimes leaning over the examining table); 2) kneeling face-down on the examining table (i.e., on all fours); or 3) lying on his side with his legs pulled up to his chest as if he were making a cannonball in diving. Then, the physician inserts a well-lubricated, gloved index finger into the anus and advances it a few inches until the prostate is felt. Normal prostate tissue has the texture of the muscle between the thumb and index finger when the two are pushed against each other, while prostate cancer feels hard like your knuckle. The prostate can sometimes have a distinct area of hardness, like a marble. This hard area is called a prostatic nodule, and is suspicious for prostate cancer.

Other findings on the DRE that raise the suspicion for prostate cancer include: induration (i.e., a cobblestone feeling of the gland), or asymmetry with one side larger or firmer than the other. Pain and tenderness during the DRE may be a sign of prostatitis. The DRE usually takes only a few seconds, and it is an essential part of the screening for prostate cancer, because even though the PSA level is more sensitive than the DRE, best of all is to do both examinations.

Laboratory Studies

Prostate Specific Antigen

Prostate specific antigen (PSA) is the most important tumor marker available for the early detection and monitoring of men with prostate cancer. PSA is a protein made almost exclusively by the prostate. It is produced by both normal and cancerous prostate cells. PSA levels can be measured with a blood test. It is normally not present in large amounts in the bloodstream. PSA levels can be elevated in patients with prostate cancer, although about 10 to 25 percent of patients with prostate cancer will have a normal PSA level. PSA can also be elevated by BPH (the bigger the gland, the more PSA it can produce) or prostatitis (inflammation in the prostate can cause blood levels of PSA to be elevated), so even though a patient's PSA level is elevated, it doesn't mean that he definitely has prostate cancer.

Other situations that may temporarily raise the PSA level include:

1. Urinary retention (see Chapter 20).
2. Ejaculation: This is controversial; however, it is suggested that PSA levels may increase up to 40 percent within one hour of ejaculation and return to baseline levels within 48 hours. Therefore, it is usually recommended that men refrain from sex for at least two days before having their PSA level checked.
3. Surgical procedures on the prostate, including TURP, biopsy of the prostate, and the minimally invasive surgical procedures, such as TUIP, TVP, TUMT, laser assisted prostatectomy, TUNA, and BDP (see Chapter 20).

Cystoscopy and catheterization of the bladder have also been shown to temporarily increase the PSA level, although some authors have reported that these two procedures do not influence the PSA result. It should be noted that Proscar (finasteride), a medication used to treat symptomatic BPH, can decrease the PSA level by 50 percent; therefore, in patients taking Proscar for three months or longer, the PSA level detected must be doubled in order to obtain their actual PSA value. As discussed in Chapter 20, alpha blockers are also medications used to treat BPH, but they have no effect on the PSA level.

There are a number of tests to measure PSA levels, and since these tests are not exactly the same, PSA results can vary slightly, depending on which brand is used and which laboratory performs the test. In general, the standard normal range for PSA values is 0 to 4 ng/ml. Studies have shown that the chance of having a biopsy positive for prostate cancer with a PSA level less than 4 ng/ml is only about 4.5 percent, whereas if the PSA level is greater than 10 ng/ml, the chance of having a positive biopsy is approximately 75 percent. When the PSA level is between 4 to 10 ng/ml, the chance of a positive biopsy is approximately 17 to 25 percent, so interpretation of this group of results is difficult. The range of PSA values (between 4 and 10 ng/ml) is called "the gray zone" by some. Various methods of interpreting PSA values have been developed in an attempt to improve the test's accuracy, and, possibly, eliminate unnecessary prostate biopsies, especially in patients with PSA levels in the gray zone.

Table 21-1: Age-Specific PSA Reference Ranges, Based on Race			
PSA Reference Ranges (ng/ml)			
Age Range (years)	Asians	Blacks	Whites
40-49	0-2.0	0-2.0	0-2.5
50-59	0-3.0	0-4.0	0-3.5
60-69	0-4.0	0-4.5	0-4.5
70-79	0-5.0	0-5.5	0-6.5

The discovery that PSA levels tend to rise with age led to the development of age-specific reference ranges. These ranges were initially based on studies in white men, and when most people discuss the age-specific PSA reference ranges, they usually mean those ranges located under "whites" in Table 21-1. Recently, it has been suggested that these age-specific reference ranges be revised to include Asian and black men, thus taking into account the slight differences in normal PSA values between the races (see Table 21-1).

The argument in favor of the age-specific reference ranges is that they increase the detection of prostate cancer in younger men (those 60 and under) and may eliminate unnecessary prostate biopsies in older men (older than 70), making PSA a more useful test for diagnosing prostate cancer. Age-specific reference ranges have not had widespread acceptance, especially since some studies have concluded that a PSA cut-off of 4.0 ng/ml was superior to all other cut-off values for all age groups. As a result, some physicians use the standard PSA range of 0 to 4 ng/ml, with any value above 4.0 being abnormal, while others believe in the age-specific reference ranges, with or without race considerations. More study needs to be done to determine the clinical significance and usefulness of the race-specific PSA reference ranges.

It has been observed that prostate cancer can lead to a ten-fold higher rise in PSA levels compared to an equal volume of BPH. As a result, the concentration of PSA in the blood can be divided by the volume of the prostate, as measured by ultrasound, in an attempt to differentiate elevation of the PSA level due to prostate cancer versus that from BPH. This diagnostic technique is called the *PSA density*. A PSA density of greater than 0.15 has been reported to be more suspicious for the presence of prostate cancer, whereas if the PSA density is less than 0.15, the source of an elevated PSA level is more likely to be BPH. In patients with a PSA value between 4 and 10 ng/ml and a PSA density greater than 0.15, there appears to be a higher risk of detecting prostate cancer, and prostate biopsy is recommended. However, since conflicting results have been published, the utility of PSA density is controversial.

The change in the PSA level over time is known as the *PSA velocity*. The currently accepted normal increase in PSA values is a maximum of 0.75 ng/ml/yr. An increase in PSA of greater than 0.75 ng/ml/yr is suspicious for the presence of prostate cancer, and it is recommended that the patient be followed more closely. For example, if the patient's DRE and PSA level are within normal limits but the PSA value increased more than 0.75 ng/ml in the past year, it is prudent to repeat the DRE and PSA level in three to six months to follow the patient more closely. If the PSA level continues to rise rapidly, or if it becomes abnormal for the patient's age, a prostate biopsy is usually recommended. Most studies indicate that for the PSA velocity to be useful, the PSA level must be checked at least three times over a period of at least two years.

PSA exists in the blood in both a "free" and "complex" form. In the complex form, PSA is bound to another protein. Most standard PSA blood tests measure the total PSA level (i.e., both the free and complex forms). Studies have shown that men with BPH have a greater amount of free PSA in their blood, whereas in men with prostate cancer, more PSA tends to be in complex form. Therefore, determining the ratio of free-to-total PSA, known as the F/T ratio, may help to differentiate prostate cancer from BPH, especially in men with total PSA levels in the 4 to 10 range. That is, the lower the F/T ratio, the greater the amount of complex PSA, and the greater the risk of prostate cancer. Initially, studies reported that if the F/T ratio was less than 0.25 (i.e., 25 percent), there was a greater chance of having a biopsy positive for cancer. Subsequent studies suggested that using a cut-off of 0.18 helped to prevent unnecessary biopsies. The general opinion today is that the F/T ratio may be useful in deciding which men need further evaluation with a prostate biopsy; however, the cut-off levels for this ratio vary between 14 and 28 percent. More study is needed to determine which cut-off level will be most accurate in differentiating between men with and without prostate cancer.

Recently, genetic engineering is being used to find even minute amounts of PSA in tissue and body fluids. More studies need to be done to determine the clinical usefulness of these techniques as well as their role in the diagnosis and management of prostate cancer.

At present, the best approach to screening men for prostate cancer appears to be the combination of the DRE and the total PSA level. For men with PSA levels in the 4 to 10 range, PSA velocity and/or the F/T ratio may be helpful in determining when prostate biopsy is indicated and, thus, help to avoid unnecessary biopsies.

Prostatic Acid Phosphatase

Acid phosphatase is an enzyme produced by a variety of body tissues; however, its highest concentrations are found in the prostate. In the past, the prostatic acid phosphatase (PAP) was measured to detect and follow prostate cancer, but since PSA has been proven to be a better method of detecting prostate cancer, the use of PAP has declined significantly. Some doctors still use PAP measurements to determine if the patient's prostate cancer has spread (i.e., in one study, 60 percent of patients with an elevated PAP were found to have lymph node metastases at the time of surgery).

Urinalysis

A urinalysis (U/A) is usually performed to check for infection, which can temporarily elevate the PSA level, and to search for other abnormalities, such as hematuria. In patients found to have a urinary tract infection, a PSA level should be delayed until a few weeks after the infection has been treated. If, however, a PSA happened to be drawn at the time of the infection and is found to be elevated, it is usually recommended that the infection be treated, and then a PSA level be repeated a few weeks after the course of treatment is complete. If the PSA level remains abnormal, further evaluation is indicated.

SPECIAL STUDIES

Transrectal Ultrasound of the Prostate

If the DRE or PSA is abnormal, further evaluation is usually recommended. During transrectal ultrasound of the prostate (TRUS), the patient lies on his side, and an ultrasound probe that is slightly larger than a person's index finger is passed into the anus and up the rectum to visualize the prostate. Ultrasound is used to detect and visualize differences between cancerous and non-cancerous prostate tissue. However, since the false negative rate of TRUS (i.e., the chance that the ultrasound will appear normal in a patient with prostate cancer) is 40 to 52 percent, most urologists feel that if the situation is suspicious enough to perform a TRUS, it is suspicious enough to perform a biopsy of the prostate, too.

Prostate Biopsy

If either the DRE or PSA level is abnormal, the chance of having a biopsy positive for prostate cancer is approximately 36 percent. If both the DRE and PSA are abnormal, the chance of a positive biopsy is 66 percent. Therefore, if either the DRE or the PSA level is abnormal, a prostate biopsy (usually with ultrasound guidance) is recommended. Biopsy of the prostate can be performed with a needle passed through the rectum using finger guidance, or with a needle passed through the perineum (the area between the scrotum and the anus). Today, prostate biopsy is usually performed with transrectal ultrasound guidance.

The night before transrectal ultrasound guided biopsy of the prostate (TRUS Bx), the patient is instructed to begin taking a prescribed antibiotic to try to decrease infectious complications after the procedure. An enema is usually prescribed to be taken in the morning of the procedure to clean out the rectum. TRUS Bx is usually performed in the office without anesthesia. The patient lies on his side with his pants off. The lubricated ultrasound probe is placed into the patient's anus and is passed gently up the rectum for one to two inches until the prostate is visualized. The size of the gland and any abnormal areas are noted. A needle is then inserted through the probe and small samples of prostate tissue are removed.

The number of biopsies that should be taken is a topic of debate. Usually three samples of tissue are taken from both sides for a total of six biopsies, but some urologists take eight or more biopsies to try to increase the chance of finding prostate cancer if it is present. The patient continues his antibiotics for one to two days after the biopsy. It is usually recommended that the patient take it easy for the rest of the day after the biopsy. The biopsies are sent to a pathologist who will examine the specimens for the presence of prostate cancer.

The overall complication rate of TRUS Bx is 2.1 percent. The risks of prostate biopsy are slight, and include:

1. Infection (0.6 percent): Although rare, if infection occurs it can cause significant problems which is why patients are prescribed antibiotics to start taking the day before the biopsy and also administer an enema to clean out the rectum on the day of the procedure. Patients with artificial

heart valves, history of valvular heart disease, or other conditions which require them to take antibiotics before dental procedures, may get additional antibiotics administered intravenously or intramuscularly to avoid infectious complications.

2. Bleeding (0.6 percent): Patients may notice some blood in their urine or with bowel movements for a few days after the biopsy. Hematospermia can be noted for up to several weeks after the biopsy. In an attempt to avoid bleeding complications, patients are usually advised to stop any aspirin products, ibuprofen (e.g., Motrin), or other blood thinners (e.g., Coumadin) for four to seven days before their biopsies.

3. Urine retention (3 percent): This problem occurs due to swelling that may develop as a result of inflammation from the biopsy; however, it is more common in patients who had voiding problems before the biopsy.

It usually takes about four to seven days for the biopsy results to return, and the three possibilities include:

• *No evidence of cancer:* This is great news, but it doesn't mean that the patient is free from follow-up. In this case, the patient is usually seen in 6 to 12 months with a repeat DRE and PSA level. If there is no significant change in either of these studies, annual DRE and PSA levels are usually recommended thereafter. If on follow-up, however, the DRE becomes suspicious or the PSA increases further, a repeat biopsy is usually recommended.

• *Atypical cells:* Sometimes, the biopsied tissue is not totally normal but isn't definitely cancerous. This condition has been called atypical hyperplasia, but is now more commonly referred to as *prostatic intraepithelial neoplasia* (PIN).

PIN is divided into three levels depending on how abnormal the cells look. Grade I (low grade PIN) has mildly abnormal cells, and grade III (high grade PIN) has severely abnormal looking cells. Grade II PIN is somewhere in between. If low grade PIN (PIN I) is found on biopsy, a follow-up DRE and PSA in three to six months is usually recommended, and if there is no significant change in these studies on follow-up, yearly follow-up DRE and PSA levels are recommended from then on. Again, if the DRE becomes abnormal or if the PSA rises further, biopsy is recommended. Studies have shown that 50 percent of patients with grade II to III PIN will have cancer found in a repeat biopsy. Therefore, if grade II to III PIN is found on biopsy, a repeat biopsy in four to six weeks is usually recommended. In those patients who, despite knowing these statistics, refuse a repeat biopsy, extremely close follow-up with a repeat DRE and PSA in three months is advised.

- *The biopsy shows cancer:* At this point, the patient will follow up with his urologist to discuss further management and treatment options. However, before deciding on treatment, the aggressiveness of the patient's cancer and whether or not it has spread outside the prostate need to be determined.

GRADE

The biopsy report usually describes the grade of the cancer. In grading, the microscopic appearance of the tumor cells is used to predict how aggressive, or fast-growing, they are. The more the tumor cells resemble normal prostatic cells, the less aggressive they are assumed to be (i.e., they are considered *well-differentiated* tumor cells), and the less the tumor cells resemble normal prostatic tissue, the more aggressive they are likely to be (i.e., they are considered *poorly differentiated* tumor cells).

There are a number of grading systems. The Gleason system is the most common grading system used today. In this system, the pathologist micro-scopically examines two areas of the tissue specimen. To each area, he assigns a grade between 1 and 5, with 1 being well-differentiated and 5 being poorly differentiated, and more likely to spread quickly. The grades from the two areas are then added together to yield a total score between 2 and 10. Therefore, a Gleason score of 2 to 4 means that the cancer appears well-differentiated and slow-growing, a score of 8 to 10 signifies a poorly differentiated tumor which is probably aggressive and rapidly growing, and a score of 5 to 7 is consistent with a moderately differentiated tumor which can be slow or fast growing. The higher the Gleason score, the more aggressive the cancer.

The other grading system, known as the Mostofi system, uses the numbers 1 to 3 to rank a tumor's aggressiveness. Well-differentiated tumors (i.e., Gleason score 2 to 4) are described as grade 1; moderately differentiated tumors (i.e., Gleason score 5 to 7) are identified as grade 2; and poorly differentiated tumors (i.e., Gleason score 8 to 10) are called grade 3 (see Table 21-2).

Table 21-2: Summary of the Grading Systems			
Pathologist Description	Aggressiveness	Mostofi Score	Gleason Score
Well differentiated	low	1	2-4
Moderately differentiated	intermediate	2	5-7
Poorly differentiated	high	3	8-10

STAGE

Stage refers to the degree of invasion or, in other words, how far the tumor has spread into the surrounding tissues or to other parts of the body, if at all. Accurate clinical staging, combined with other clinical data available at diagnosis, helps the urologist assess the prognosis of the patient and make rational treatment recommendations. There are two staging systems in common use. The first is the original ABCD system of Whitmore, modified by Jewett (so now it's called the Whitmore-Jewett System), and the second is the more recent international TNM classification, which stands for T - tumor, N - nodes (i.e., lymph node involvement), and M - metastases (i.e., distant spread of cancer).

The Whitmore-Jewett System

- **Stage A** is microscopic disease found incidentally in 10 to 20 percent of patients after TURP or open prostatectomy for symptomatic BPH. DRE is normal.
  - A1 is focal disease with tumor found in 5 percent or less of tissue resected.
  - A2 is diffuse disease with tumor found in more than 5 percent of tissue resected.

- Ax is cancer diagnosed as a result of an elevated PSA (some call this B0).
- **Stage B** is gross disease palpable on DRE believed to be confined to the prostate.
    - B1 is a single nodule or induration involving half of one side (or lobe) or less.
    - B2 is induration of one or both lobes.
- **Stage C** describes tumor extending locally beyond the prostate without metastatic disease.
    - C1 is minimal extraprostatic extension without involvement of the seminal vesicles.
    - C2 is extensive extraprostatic spread with involvement of 1 or both seminal vesicles.
- **Stage D** is metastatic disease with cancer spread far beyond the prostate.
    - D0 is clinically localized cancer (A, B, or C) with an elevated PAP suggesting undetected metastatic cancer.
    - D1 denotes patients with cancer involving the lymph nodes around the prostate.
    - D2 describes patients with cancer spread to bone or other distant organs.
    - D3 is used to denote patients with metastatic disease who relapse after hormone therapy.

The TNM Classification

- **T1** is tumor found incidentally after another procedure, such as TURP. DRE is normal.
    - T1a is focal disease with tumor found in 5 percent or less of tissue resected.
    - T1b is diffuse disease with tumor found in more than 5 percent of tissue resected.
    - T1c denotes patients with nonpalpable tumor identified because of an elevated PSA level.

- **T2** is clinically palpable tumor confined to the prostate.
    - T2a describes a cancer that occupies half of a lobe or less.
    - T2b is a cancer that involves more than half of a lobe but not both lobes.
    - T2c is a cancer that occupies any percentage of both prostate lobes.
- **T3** involves tumor outside the prostate.
    - T3a is extraprostatic spread on one side of the gland.
    - T3b is extraprostatic spread on both sides of the gland.
    - T3c is extraprostatic spread involving one or both seminal vesicles.
- **T4** involves extensive local tumor spread outside the prostate invading the bladder neck, rectum, or other adjacent structures.
    - T4a is a cancer that has spread to the bladder neck, external sphincter, or rectum.
    - T4b is a cancer that invades the pelvic muscles or pelvic side wall.
- **N0** signifies that no lymph nodes near the prostate have been invaded by cancer.
- **N1** denotes that cancer has spread to one lymph node (2 cm or smaller).
- **N2** describes when the cancer has spread to one lymph node 2 to 5 cm, or to multiple lymph nodes, all totaling less than 5 cm in size.
- **N3** signifies that cancer in the lymph nodes has achieved a size of 5 cm or larger.
- **M0** signifies that the cancer has not spread far beyond the prostate or local lymph nodes.
- **M1** indicates that the cancer has spread far beyond the prostate (e.g., to the bones, liver, or lungs).

Therefore, if the TNM system is used to stage a patient's prostate cancer, three areas are addressed (i.e., the tumor, lymph nodes, and the presence of metastatic disease). A comparison of the two staging systems is seen in Table 21-3.

The most accurate method to determine the stage of the patient's prostate cancer is to surgically remove the gland and local lymph nodes and examine them microscopically, thus determining the pathologic stage of disease. However, a variety of "non-invasive" tests have also been used to estimate the clinical stage of the patient's cancer and to help guide treatment recommendations. Some staging studies that may be used include:

- *Computed axial tomography scan (CT scan):* This is an x-ray study during which the patient lies down on a table which is passed through a circular machine that, with the help of a computer, makes cross-sectional images of the body. It is used to search for enlarged lymph nodes around the prostate, or for evidence of metastatic disease. Since an iodine-based contrast solution is administered intravenously to help visualize certain structures, the risks of CT scan are similar to those for IVP (see Chapter 18). The false negative rate of CT scan is 40 to 50 percent (which means it may be read as normal in up to 50 percent of patients with disease outside the prostate). Therefore, CT scan is usually not recommended unless the PSA level is greater than 20 ng/ml.

- *Magnetic resonance imaging scan (MRI):* This study requires that the patient lie still for 30 to 40 minutes in a tube-shaped chamber that uses magnetic waves, instead of x-rays, to take pictures of the patient's internal organs. The chamber of the MRI machine is so small that patients who are claustrophobic may not be able to tolerate it for the time required to complete the scan. Since the false negative rate of MRI is similar to that for CT scan, it is also usually not recommended unless the patient's PSA level is greater than 20 ng/ml.

Table 21-3: Summary of the TNM and Whitmore-Jewett Staging Systems

TNM	WJ	What the Results Mean
T0	-	No cancer.
T1a	A1	Incidental finding of cancer after treatment for BPH. The cancer occupies 5% or less of the tissue resected.
T1b	A2	Incidental finding but the cancer occupies more than 5% of the tissue resected. Cancer not detected byDRE or PSA.
T1c	Ax (B0)	A cancer that cannot be felt with DRE but is detected due to an elevated PSA level.
T2a	B1	A cancer that is palpable on DRE and occupies 50% or less of one prostatic lobe.
T2b	B1	A cancer that occupies more than 50% of one prostatic lobe.
T2c	B2	A cancer that involves both lobes of the prostate.
T3a	C1	Extraprostatic spread on one side of the prostate.
T3b	C1	Extraprostatic spread on both sides of the prostate.
T3c	C2	Extraprostatic spread to one or both seminal vesicles.
T4a	C2	Extraprostatic spread involving the bladder neck, external sphincter, and/or rectum.
T4b	C2	Extraprostatic spread invading other areas near the prostate.
N0	-	No lymph nodes have been invaded by cancer.
N1	D1	A cancer has spread to one lymph node 2 cm. or smaller.
N2	D1	A cancer has spread to one lymph node between 2-5 cm. in size, or to multiple lymph nodes totaling less than 5 cm. in size.
N3	D1	Cancer in the lymph nodes has achieved a size of > 5 cm.
M0	-	No distant metastases.
M1	D2	The cancer has spread far beyond the prostate (e.g., to bones, liver, or lungs.

Modified from: Oesterling, JE and Moyad, MA, *The ABC's of Prostate Cancer*. Lanham, MD: Madison Books, 1997.

- *Bone scan:* Since the second most common place that prostate cancer spreads to once it gets outside the prostate is the patient's bones, a bone scan is sometimes used to find advanced (metastatic) prostate cancer. In this test, a radioactive solution is injected intravenously. This nuclear material, or tracer, is taken up by areas of bone that are trying to regenerate. Areas of bone to which prostate cancer has spread will concentrate the nuclear tracer, and this will show up on a machine that searches for radioactivity. Other conditions that can cause bone to accumulate the radioactive tracer include: arthritis, old fractures, or infections in the bone. Studies have shown that if the PSA level is less than 10 ng/ml, the chance of having a positive bone scan (i.e., one that is suggestive of prostate cancer metastatic to bone) is minimal. As a result, most urologists no longer recommend a bone scan in patients with recently diagnosed prostate cancer who have a PSA level less than 10 ng/ml and no symptoms of bone pain. However, some urologists still like to obtain a baseline bone scan to have something to compare future studies to if a patient's symptoms change or if his disease appears to be progressing, such as would be the case if the PSA level starts to rise.

- *Pelvic lymph node dissection (PLND):* The most common place that prostate cancer usually spreads to when it gets outside the prostate is to the lymph nodes surrounding the prostate. PLND is a surgical procedure in which the lymph nodes around the prostate are sampled in an attempt to stage the patient. This procedure can be performed in one of two ways:

  - *Laparoscopic PLND:* Under general anesthesia, a telescopic instrument is passed into the abdomen through a puncture site near the belly-button. Then, surgical instruments are placed through several other puncture sites in the lower abdomen to remove lymph nodes that will be examined by the pathologist for the presence of cancer cells. The operation takes about one or two hours, depending on the experience of the urologist, and the patient usually goes home on the day of surgery or the following morning.

  - *Open PLND:* With the patient under general or spinal anesthesia, the urologist makes an incision in the lower abdomen, and removes the pelvic lymph nodes around the prostate. The lymph nodes are then examined by the pathologist for the presence of cancer cells. If prostate cancer is found in the lymph nodes, the incision is closed, and treatment options for advanced prostate cancer are subsequently discussed with the patient. If no evidence of cancer is found in the lymph nodes, surgery to remove the prostate gland may still be an option. Therefore, if the patient is a candidate for surgery and has decided on surgical removal of the prostate to treat his prostate cancer, open PLND can usually be carried out immediately before the prostatectomy under the same anesthesia.

Table 21-4 indicates that the higher the PSA level, the greater the risk that the patient's prostate cancer has spread to the lymph nodes. Some studies have suggested that PLND need not be performed if the PSA level is less than 10 ng/ml and the tumor grade on biopsy is well or moderately well differentiated (i.e., Gleason score of 7 or less), since, in these instances, the risk of spread to the lymph nodes is minimal (2 to 5 percent). If, however, the PSA level is greater than 10 ng/ml, or if the patient has high grade tumor on biopsy, then a PLND is usually recommended before proceeding with surgical removal of the prostate.

Table 21-4: Risk of Prostate Cancer Spread to Lymph Nodes Based on PSA	
PSA (ng/ml)	Likelihood of + PLND
0-3.9	2.0%
4-9.9	5.3%
10-19.9	13.2%
>20	29.5%
>50	47.3%

- *Radioimmunologic imaging.* Antibodies are proteins that help the body fight infection by recognizing and binding to foreign substances. In the laboratory, antibodies to PSA have been made, and these antibodies can be joined to radioactive substances. These radioactive "tagged" antibodies to PSA can then be utilized to permit identification and imaging of tumor in metastatic sites. Early results of these experiments are encouraging, but more study is needed to determine the indications and ultimate usefulness of this diagnostic modality.

The DRE, PSA level, and grade of the biopsy specimen based on the Gleason score can help to clinically stage a patient's prostate cancer, so many of the above studies are not routinely used in staging. Once the patient's PSA level and tumor grade are determined and the clinical stage is estimated, the urologist usually discusses the various treatment options available and makes recommendations for the treatment of the patient's cancer. These recommendations are based on many pieces of information, some of which include: the age and general health of the patient, the likelihood that the cancer is confined to the prostate, and the information regarding the various treatment options available at the present time. The patient is usually given some time to think about his options, and to even seek a second opinion if he chooses, before making a final decision as to how he wants his prostate cancer to be treated.

TREATMENT OPTIONS

Surgery

Radical prostatectomy involves the surgical removal of the prostate, seminal vesicles, and a piece of both vas deferens in an attempt to definitively treat prostate cancer. Before surgery, there are a few steps that are usually taken to optimize conditions for the procedure:

1. It is usually recommended to wait six weeks from the time of the prostate biopsy before performing surgery to allow the area between the rectum and the prostate to heal adequately. After TURP, it is recommended that the patient wait 12 weeks before proceeding with radical prostatectomy.

2. It is recommended that the patient stop using aspirin, ibuprofen, or other products that can thin their blood for at least one week before surgery to prevent excessive bleeding during or after the procedure.

3. Since some patients lose enough blood to require a blood transfusion during or after their surgery, in the weeks before radical prostatectomy, patients may be asked to donate their own blood for the specific purpose of having it available in case they need a transfusion during or after the operation. This is called *autologous blood donation.*

4. The patient is usually given a laxative to clear out his intestines on the day before his surgery and is advised not to eat or drink anything after midnight the night before surgery. The patient may also receive an enema to clean out the rectum in the hospital on the morning of his surgery.

There are two basic ways that a radical prostatectomy can be performed depending on the incision that is used. The approach chosen is a matter of training, surgical expertise, and personal preference.

Radical Retropubic Prostatectomy

Most urologists are familiar with and have been trained with this approach. In fact, it accounts for 85 percent of all radical prostatectomies. The patient is usually admitted on the day of surgery. This procedure can be performed under general anesthesia, a special type of spinal anesthesia called epidural anesthesia, or some combination of these two. With the patient lying flat, a vertical incision is made from just below the belly-button to just above the penis. If indicated, a PLND is performed first. If the prostate cancer is found to have spread to the lymph nodes, it is generally believed that surgery to remove the prostate will not help the patient live longer, so the patient is usually closed up and other treatment options are explored. If it appears that the cancer is confined to the prostate, the prostate is cut away from the urethra and the prostate is cut away from the bladder. The prostate, seminal vesicles, and part of each vas deferens are removed and sent to the pathologist for examination and pathologic staging, and the bladder is sewn to the urethra (see Figure 21-1).

The nerves and blood vessels responsible for erections run along the posterior aspect of both sides of the prostate. Thanks to the development of the technique by Dr. Patrick Walsh of John's Hopkins Hospital, these nerves can sometimes be dissected away from the prostate and spared in an attempt

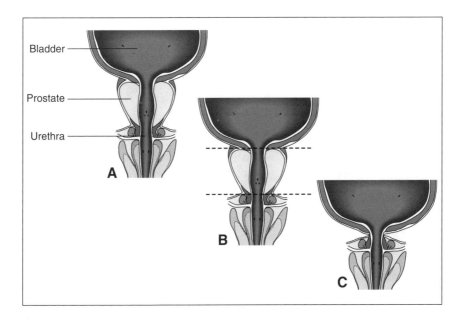

Figure 21-1: *Radical Prostatectomy: A) Schematic drawing of the lower urinary tract; B) The prostate is cut away from the urethra and bladder (----- marks the sites of transection); C) The bladder is sewn to the urethra.*

to preserve sexual function in patients undergoing radical prostatectomy. The procedure is called the nerve-sparing approach. There are certain contraindications to the nerve-sparing procedure, and these situations include:

- If the patient is impotent already, there is no benefit to sparing the nerves.

- If the prostate feels hard on one side before or during surgery, it is recommended that the nerves not be spared on that side.

- If the nerves are adherent to the prostate during surgery, it is recommended to remove them with the specimen.

- It is recommended to not spare the nerves on the side of a positive biopsy; therefore, if cancer is found on biopsies from both sides, some studies recommend not sparing the nerves on either side. It should be noted that even though an attempt is made to spare the nerves, there are no guarantees that this part of the operation will be a success.

A catheter is passed through the urethra into the bladder for urine drainage at the end of the procedure. The operation generally lasts about two to three hours. The patient usually starts taking fluids by mouth on the day after surgery, and may start eating a regular diet on the second or third post-operative day. The patient usually spends three to five days in the hospital, after which he is discharged home with pain medications and with the catheter hooked to a drainage bag which wraps around the patient's leg to allow him to wear pants. The catheter is left in place for two to three weeks to allow the area where the bladder is sewn to the urethra to heal. The patient returns to the office to have his catheter removed and his PSA level checked. After a radical prostatectomy, a normal PSA level is anything less than 0.5 ng/ml. The patient is advised to avoid strenuous activity and lifting heavy objects for four to six weeks after surgery to allow ample time for the wound to heal and to avoid developing a hernia. He is also advised not to drive for one to two weeks. Walking, however, is encouraged.

Although radical prostatectomy is considered the most effective treatment for patients with organ-confined prostate cancer, many people fear it because of its associated morbidity. There are also a number of complications that have been reported after radical prostatectomy:

1. Infection (1 percent).

2. Bleeding: Average blood loss during the operation is between 500 and 1000 cc. The risk that the patient will need to have more surgery for bleeding is approximately 0.1 percent. Approximately 10 percent of patients will need a blood transfusion during or after their surgery, and this is when autologous blood may be used. In addition, now there are machines that allow surgeons to collect blood that is lost during surgery. After processing, this blood can be given back to the patient. Even with all these precautions, there is still a very rare possibility that the patient may lose enough blood to require a transfusion from the blood bank. Because blood is now screened for hepatitis and AIDS, any risks associated with banked blood are low.

3. Pain: This is major surgery, but post-operatively, various medications are used to control the patient's pain and keep him as comfortable as

possible. Patients are also given a prescription for oral pain medication to take at home as needed for two to three weeks after their surgery.

4. Hernia: Weaknesses can develop in the area of the incision or in the groin area after radical retropubic prostatectomy. For this reason, patients are advised not to perform any strenuous activity and to avoid lifting anything heavier than 5 to 10 lb. for four to six weeks after surgery.

5. Lymphocele (0.4 to 2.3 percent): Sometimes after PLND, lymph fluid can leak out of lymph vessels and form a collection which is called a lymphocele. Patients with this problem can present with a mass or pain in the lower abdomen, which can be diagnosed with ultrasound or CT scan. Symptomatic lymphoceles are usually treated by needle aspiration of the fluid, but rarely, surgery may be necessary to prevent recurrences. In an attempt to prevent fluid collections after radical retropubic prostatectomy, a drain is usually placed in the pelvis and brought out through a small incision in the lower abdomen. It is usually removed in two to four days when drainage ceases (this is different from the urinary drainage catheter that exits the penis and is left in place for two to three weeks).

6. Rectal injury (0.1 to 1.0 percent): The rectum is located immediately posterior to the prostate. In fact, as explained in the section on prostate biopsy, biopsies of the prostate are usually taken by going through the rectal wall. Occasionally, a hole or tear can occur in the rectum during radical prostatectomy. If the hole is small, it can be sewn closed, and if the patient is kept on antibiotics for a while most of the time, no significant sequelae occur. If it's a large hole, or if the patient has had prior radiation therapy to this area, a temporary colostomy may be necessary to allow adequate healing.

7. Ureteral injury (1 percent): This rare problem is usually detected during the operation and can be repaired at that time.

8. Damage to adjacent structures: Other structures, such as the intestines or blood vessels may occasionally be injured during this surgery.

9. Deep vein thrombosis (1 to 2 percent) and/or pulmonary embolus (1 to 2 percent): During this procedure, patients lie on the operating table for

two to three hours while the urologist operates around blood vessels in the pelvis. As a result, clots can form in the veins that drain the legs (i.e., a condition called deep vein thrombosis, or DVT). Symptoms of DVT include asymmetric swelling or pain in the legs, but DVT can be present without symptoms. Sometimes, too, these clots can break free and travel through the bloodstream to lodge in the lungs, causing a potentially fatal condition known as pulmonary embolus, or PE. Symptoms of PE include fever, shortness of breathe, or rapid heart rate. Some steps that may be taken to try to decrease the risk of DVT or PE include a) the use of special compression stockings that massage the patient's legs to keep the blood moving while he's on the operating table and in bed after surgery, b) trying to get the patient to move his legs and ambulate as soon as possible after the operation, and c) the occasional use of blood thinners for a short time after surgery.

10. Urine leak: Sometimes, it may take longer than usual for the bladder and urethra to heal together. This problem usually resolves by keeping the urinary catheter in place for a longer period of time.

11. Anastomotic stricture (1 to 22 percent): The area where the bladder is sewn to the urethra is known as the *urethrovesical anastomosis*. When two tubes of tissue in the body are sewn together, extra scar tissue can develop with healing. If extra scar tissue develops at the urethrovesical anastomosis, the condition, known as an anastomotic stricture, can result in difficulty voiding. This problem may be treated by placing progressively larger metal rods up the urethra to dilate the area of scar tissue (50 percent success rate), or may require surgery to cut away the scar tissue (approximately 60 percent success rate).

12. Impotence: If the nerves to the penis are not spared, the chance of having normal erections is almost zero. If the nerves are spared on one side, the chance of being able to have an erection adequate for intercourse has been reported to be approximately 40 percent, and if the nerves are spared on both sides, the chance of having adequate erections has been reported to be between 60 and 70 percent. The best chance of preserving sexual function if the nerves are spared occurs in men less than 60 years of age with small tumors. Yet, it can take up to one year after surgery

for sexual function to return, if at all. Fortunately, even if impotence does occur after radical prostatectomy, there are many successful treatment options available today to help patients improve their sex life (see Chapter 6). Given the overall results with the nerve-sparing approach, combined with the treatment options available, erectile dysfunction should be less of a concern when deciding on the most appropriate therapy for clinically localized prostate cancer.

13. Incontinence (0.5 to 35 percent): Total incontinence with almost constant leakage occurs in up to 17 percent of patients, and leakage only during strenuous activity can occur in up to 35 percent of patients. However, improved techniques have significantly reduced the rate of incontinence after radical prostatectomy. Usually, patients start noting that they achieve dryness at night, then, they note that they achieve dryness when walking, and finally, when performing strenuous activity. The urologist may teach his patients certain exercises that can be done after surgery to strengthen some of the muscles used for continence. Approximately 50 percent of patients are continent by three months after the operation, 80 percent are "dry" by six months, and 90 percent are continent by one year. The age of the patient appears to affect continence rates since the results are better in patients under 60 years old. There are a number of successful treatment alternatives for those rare patients with significant leakage that persists one year after surgery.

14. Residual or recurrent tumor: After surgery, the specimen is sent to a pathologist who examines the prostate and seminal vesicles to try to determine if all of the cancer has been removed. If all the margins of resection are free of tumor and the cancer does not appear to have gotten outside the prostate, no further treatment is usually recommended, except routine follow-up visits, since the chance of tumor recurrence (as might be evidenced by a rising PSA) is only approximately 9 to 14 percent. The patient just requires routine follow-up DRE and PSA levels every 6 to 12 months for a few years to be sure that his DRE remains normal and his PSA level stays less than 0.5 ng/ml. If the PSA level starts to rise or if DRE reveals the patient has developed nodularity

where his prostate was, it could signal a recurrence of his prostate cancer from tumor cells left behind, because they were too small to be seen or felt at the time of the initial surgery. Sometimes, the pathology report reveals that cancer cells extend up to, and thus beyond, the margins of resection (indicating that tumor was left behind). What to do next is a controversial issue, but along with the presence or absence of positive margins, the grade of the tumor needs to be considered as well. Some studies suggest that if the margins are positive but the Gleason score is less than 8 (indicating that the tumor is not high grade), only close follow-up is needed unless the PSA level should start to rise. If, however, the patient has both positive margins and a high grade tumor, additional radiation therapy should be carried out.

15. Possibility of finding no residual cancer in the specimen: This is a rare situation but may occur in any operation where a prior biopsy showed an area of cancer. The chance of this situation occurring is lower if more than one core obtained during the prostate biopsy shows cancer.

16. Heart attack and death (0.2 to 0.6 percent): Because of current operative techniques and perioperative care, in addition to the fact that patients are required to be in such good health to be candidates for this surgery, these complications are rare occurrences.

The results of radical prostatectomy show it to have the best 15-year survival rates of all the treatment options. It can cure prostate cancer. So, although it is associated with a lot of potential risks, the benefits of surgery probably outweigh the risks in men who are expected to live ten years more or longer (especially those under 70 who are in good health) and whose cancer is believed to be confined to the prostate. Radical prostatectomy is probably not a good choice for:

• Men whose life expectancy is less than ten years.

• Men with other serious medical conditions, such as coronary artery disease or congestive heart failure.

• Men whose prostate cancer appears to be outside the prostate at the time of diagnosis.

Radical Perineal Prostatectomy

A second type of prostate surgery is radical perineal prostatectomy. The patient is typically admitted on the day of surgery, and the operation is usually performed under general anesthesia. The patient is positioned on his back with his legs up in special stirrups to allow access to the perineum, the area between the scrotum and the anus. A semicircular incision is made between the anal opening and the scrotum. Once the prostate is exposed, the prostate, seminal vesicles, and pieces of the vas deferens are removed, and the bladder is then sewn to the urethra as in the retropubic approach. The perineal approach is better for obese men. Patients tend to have less post-operative pain and less bleeding with perineal prostatectomy as opposed to the retropubic approach.

The disadvantages of the perineal approach versus the retropubic approach include: 1) it is more difficult to perform a nerve-sparing procedure; 2) it has a higher risk of rectal injury; and 3) if a PLND is indicated, it must be performed using either laparoscopy or a separate incision in the lower abdomen. Other than the differences discussed above, the risks and success rates for radical perineal prostatectomy are similar to those of radical retropubic prostatectomy.

Radiation Therapy

External-beam Radiation Therapy

In this procedure, the patient lies on a table, and a machine focuses x-ray beams on the prostate and local lymph nodes to destroy cancer cells. Lead is used to shield other areas of the body. Each treatment lasts 15 to 30 minutes. External radiation therapy usually comprises five sessions per week for seven weeks, for a total of 35 treatment sessions. After this, the patient is followed by his urologist with a DRE and PSA level every six to twelve months.

The risks of external radiation therapy include:

1. Impotence (30 to 50 percent): Up to 50 percent of patients can experience erectile difficulty after treatment, although it may take some time for this problem to develop.

2. Gastrointestinal problems (30 to 40 percent during treatment but 10 percent long-term): Diarrhea, rectal pain and bleeding, and the urge to have a bowel movement are common due to the inflammation that results during the treatment phase. These symptoms usually resolve after the course of treatment is complete; however, 5 to 10 percent of patients may experience chronic bowel symptoms after radiation therapy.

3. Urinary problems (10 percent): Patients undergoing external radiation therapy may experience irritative voiding symptoms, such as frequency, urgency, and dysuria. These symptoms usually resolve after the treatment course is complete. The risk of scar tissue, or stricture, formation in the urethra is small, but to avoid this problem, it is usually recommended that radiation therapy be delayed 8 to 12 weeks after a TURP or other prostate surgery. Incontinence is rare after radiation therapy (less than 3 percent), but radiation can damage blood vessels supplying the bladder. As a result, even many years after radiation therapy, the lining of the bladder can become friable and may bleed easily, causing intermittent episodes of hematuria (2 to 20 percent).

Up to ten years after treatment, the survival outcomes for patients with localized prostate cancer treated with external-beam radiation therapy are similar to those treated with radical prostatectomy. However, beyond ten years after treatment, there are slightly lower success rates in the radiation-treated patients. It should be noted that in the first year after radiation therapy, the PSA level falls in 80 percent of patients, but after that first year, it continues to fall in only 8 percent of patients. In fact, studies have shown that approximately 50 to 80 percent of patients will note a rise in their PSA level three to five years after completing external radiation therapy.

External radiation therapy can be used for men of any age with any stage of prostate cancer, but the best candidates for this form of treatment include:

• Men who are expected to live at least ten more years.
• Men whose cancer is confined to the prostate.

- Men who cannot be cured by surgery, such as those whose cancer is believed to be locally outside the prostate at the time of diagnosis or those whose cancer returns after surgical treatment.
- Men who do not want to be treated with surgery.
- Men who are not candidates for surgery due to health reasons (e.g., coronary artery disease).

Radioactive Seed Implants (Interstitial Radiotherapy or Brachytherapy)

In this form of treatment, radioactive pellets (called seeds), made of iodine, palladium, or gold are placed inside the prostate, usually via the perineal approach. The seeds give off radiation which destroys cancer cells in the prostate. These seeds are usually left in place permanently; however, there is also a procedure in which radioactive seeds of iridium are placed into the prostate, the treatment administered and then the seeds are removed after approximately one and a half hours.

Patients to receive radioactive seed implants are told to abstain from aspirin or other blood thinners for at least one week before the procedure. An enema is administered on the day of the operation to clean out the rectum. The size and location of the patient's prostate, ascertained by a combination of x-rays and ultrasound, help to determine how many seeds will be placed. Under spinal anesthesia, between 70 to 150 radioactive seeds are implanted into the prostate using needles passed through the perineum with ultrasound guidance. The procedure usually lasts 30 to 60 minutes, and a catheter is placed for urinary drainage until the spinal anesthesia wears off. The patient is advised to avoid driving for 24 hours and to avoid strenuous activity for two to three days. The radioactivity of the seeds diminishes over time and is usually gone by one year. Although this radiation is not believed to travel beyond the prostate, it is generally recommended that pregnant women and children stay at least six feet away from patients with these implants for the first few months after the procedure.

Brachytherapy tends to be well tolerated with an overall complication rate of 10 to 25 percent. Some of the risks include: 1) rectal irritation and proctitis (5 to 20 percent); and 2) urinary tract symptoms (10 to 37 percent).

Irritative symptoms, such as frequency and dysuria may take a while to resolve completely. Incontinence has been reported in up to 15 percent of patients who had undergone a prior TURP, but is almost non-existent in those patients without prior prostatic surgery. Some investigators believe that radiation seed implants result in a lower incidence of impotence than external radiation therapy; but several studies have reported impotence rates of 25 to 61 percent with brachytherapy.

The results of seed implants done in the 1970s were not very good, and this technique fell into disfavor. It has been hypothesized that with today's better technology and better understanding of prostate cancer, seed therapy results will improve. Initial five-year data suggest that modern brachytherapy is equivalent to external radiation therapy in the short-term, but longer follow-up of 10 to 15 years is required to determine the true efficacy and ultimate role of this treatment option.

Presently, brachytherapy is a viable option for the following patients:

- Men with localized prostate cancer who have a life expectancy of at least ten years.
- Men older than 70 years of age with localized prostate cancer who are not candidates for surgery due to other medical problems.
- Men with clinically localized prostate cancer who do not want surgery to treat their cancer.

It is probably not a good choice for men with a significant amount of disease outside the prostate.

Cryotherapy

Cryotherapy is an experimental procedure which involves freezing the prostate in an attempt to destroy cancer cells. Patients are given an enema to clean out the rectum the night before surgery. The procedure is usually performed under general or spinal anesthesia. Transrectal ultrasound is performed to visualize the prostate and guide needle placement. Metallic needles are then passed through the perineum and into the prostate. Liquid nitrogen is infused through these needles to freeze the prostate and destroy cancer cells. A special warming device is used to prevent freezing and damage to the urethra. The procedure takes approximately two hours, and patients are usually sent home the day of the operation or the following morning with antibiotics and pain medication. Since this procedure causes inflammation and swelling of the prostate, a catheter for urinary drainage may be required for a few weeks until the swelling resolves. After the surgery, patients are monitored with regular DRE and PSA level.

There are several complications associated with cryotherapy, including:

1. Infection (20 percent): This problem has been diminished with the use of prophylactic antibiotics.

2. Pain (less than 5 percent): Patients may experience discomfort in the perineal area for a few days after the procedure, but the risk of long-term perineal pain is rare.

3. Fistula formation (0 to 4 percent): A fistula is a connection between two organs, and in this case the fistula tends to occur between the rectum and the urethra which can result in significant infections and will usually require surgery to repair.

4. Passage of prostatic tissue during voiding (2 to 19 percent): As the frozen prostatic tissue dies, it sloughs (peels off or falls away from the remaining viable tissue) and can be noted to pass during urination. It may block up the urethra which occasionally requires surgery, similar to a TURP, to open up the urethra.

5. Urethral stricture (1 to 2 percent): Scarring can occur if the urethra is damaged by exposure to the cold temperatures used in this procedure. Use of the urethral warming device has helped to minimize this problem.

6. Impotence (41 to 86 percent).

There have not been any deaths reported from cryotherapy.

So far, cryotherapy has been used to treat patients who have failed radiation therapy or in experimental protocols in patients who are not candidates for, or who do not want, surgery or radiation therapy. It is an experimental procedure and most of the studies currently evaluating this modality are carried out at university medical centers. Cryotherapy's long-term effectiveness and side effects and its ultimate role in the management of prostate cancer are yet to be determined.

Hormone Therapy

Normal metabolic functions of prostate cells require testosterone and dihydrotestosterone. These proteins are some of the male hormones called androgens. Testosterone is the major circulating androgen in the body. Ninety percent of all testosterone is produced by the testicles, and 10 percent comes from the adrenal glands, which are a pair of small glands located just above each kidney. Prostate cancer is made up of cells that require androgens for some of their metabolic functions and cells that do not need androgens to function. If deprived of testosterone, 80 percent of prostate cancers will atrophy and go into remission for a certain period of time. Therefore, hormone therapy is not a cure, but it is used to increase the length and improve the quality of life. As a result, hormone therapy is generally reserved for patients whose prostate cancer has spread outside the prostate.

There are various methods of decreasing the body's testosterone levels.

Bilateral Orchiectomy

In this operation, which is usually performed as an outpatient procedure under general or spinal anesthesia, an incision is made in the scrotum (i.e., the sac that contains the testicles), and both testicles are surgically removed. The testosterone level in the body diminishes to almost zero within three to four hours (remember that about 10 percent of the body's testosterone is supplied by the adrenal glands). Patients are instructed to keep the incision dry for two to three days, but they can usually resume normal daily activities on the day after surgery.

Unfortunately, there are several unavoidable side effects of bilateral orchiectomy. These and other possible side effects include the following:

1. Impotence (approximately 100 percent).
2. Decreased sex drive (100 percent).
3. Hot flashes (50 to 60 percent).
4. Breast enlargement or nipple sensitivity (50 percent): This can be prevented with low-dose radiation to the breast area administered a few days before beginning hormone therapy.
5. Weight gain (90 percent).
6. Decreased energy level (due to decreased testosterone levels).

Estrogen Therapy

This group of proteins is also known as the female hormones. The most commonly used in prostate cancer is diethylstilbestrol (DES). DES can result in castrate levels of testosterone in about two weeks through its effect on the pituitary gland. It is one of the most cost-effective options for the hormonal treatment of metastatic prostate cancer, but it fell into disfavor due to significant cardiovascular side effects at higher doses. The other side effects of DES are similar to those of bilateral orchiectomy.

Luteinizing Hormone Releasing Hormone (LHRH) Agonists

LHRH agonists (e.g., Lupron and Zoladex) are given by injection and, after initially stimulating an increase in testosterone levels in the week after the first injection (a condition known as the "flare phenomenon"), subsequently result in decreased testosterone levels in about two weeks. These medications exert their effect by influencing the pituitary gland. Patients who chose hormone treatment with LHRH agonists were initially required to return to their urologist every month for another injection, since the effect of these injections wore off in about one month. Now, there are longer-acting injections that can last three or four months. The indications and side effects of LHRH agonists are the same as those for bilateral orchiectomy, except that it is also possible to have an allergic reaction to these medications.

The disadvantages of LHRH agonists include:

1. They may require additional medications at the beginning of treatment to prevent tumor flare.
2. They require trips to the doctor every three to four months just for the injection for the rest of the patient's life (unless the patient subsequently decides to undergo a bilateral orchiectomy).
3. The injections are extremely expensive (about $500/month).

It appears that although bilateral orchiectomy is simple, well-tolerated, and cost-effective, the psychological effect of orchiectomy, perceived by some as a loss of manhood, cannot be underestimated. When given a choice, most men opt for LHRH agonists over orchiectomy, despite the cost.

Antiandrogens

These are drugs that block the effect of testosterone by preventing it from interacting with cancer cells. Some antiandrogens include: flutamide (Eulexin), bicalutamide (Casodex), nilutamide (Nilandron), cyproterone acetate, and ketoconazole. Commonly reported side effects of antiandrogens include: diarrhea (10 to 20 percent) (especially with flutamide); constipation (10 to 20 percent); liver problems (2 percent); nausea and vomiting. Nilutamide has been shown to cause lung inflammation in less than 2 percent of patients and may also result in a mild form of night blindness.

For complete effectiveness, antiandrogens must be used in combination with either bilateral orchiectomy or LHRH agonists. The combined use of bilateral orchiectomy (or LHRH agonists) and antiandrogens, known as combination therapy or pan androgen suppression, is designed to eliminate the 90 percent of testosterone produced by the testicles and to block the effect of the remaining 10 percent of testosterone produced by the adrenal glands. Some studies have shown that patients treated with combination therapy live a few months longer than those treated with bilateral orchiectomy or LHRH agonists alone. Antiandrogens are also very expensive (about $250/month), and many patients choose not to add antiandrogens to their treatment regimen early on for financial reasons.

Hormone therapy has been suggested for a short period of time (e.g., three to six months) before radical prostatectomy or radiation therapy to decrease the size of the cancer and possibly improve long-term success rates. This technique is known as neoadjuvant hormone therapy and is controversial. Although neoadjuvant hormone therapy for three months prior to radical surgery may decrease the prostate size in men with extremely large prostates, thus facilitating surgery, longer follow-up studies are needed to determine whether neoadjuvant hormone therapy offers a significant survival advantage over surgery or radiation therapy alone.

The problem with hormone therapy is that it only works on the population of prostate cancer cells that are hormone-sensitive (which accounts for about 80 percent of tumor cells initially). The hormone-resistant cancer cells continue to grow and proliferate, and eventually hormone therapy is no longer effective, as evidenced by a subsequent rise in PSA level. Although every patient is different, on average, hormone therapy is effective for about two to eight years before PSA levels start to rise again.

Recently, some studies have tried to use hormone therapy intermittently. This means that the patient receives an LHRH agonist, with or without an antiandrogen, until his PSA level becomes almost undetectable. Then, the patient is followed with regular DRE and PSA levels, and no more hormone therapy is administered until the PSA level starts to rise, signaling disease progression. At that point, hormone therapy is re-instituted until the PSA level again becomes almost undetectable, and the "cycle" continues. Studies in animals suggested that similar "hormone cycling" might prolong threefold to fourfold the time to emergence of the androgen-independent cells. Intermittent hormone therapy is still in the experimental stage, and clinical trials are currently underway to determine the validity of this hypothesis.

Chemotherapy

If hormone therapy fails, other drug treatments, such as chemotherapy, can be tried. To date, however, overall results from chemotherapeutic trials have been disappointing, with 10 percent response rates and response duration of about six months. Intense research in this area is producing newer agents that are being evaluated in clinical protocols at various cancer centers throughout the United States. No effective agent is available yet, however.

Watchful Waiting

Even if they choose not to receive any definitive therapy, some patients with prostate cancer will live five to ten years or longer. The realization of this fact has led to the treatment option called watchful waiting, also known as surveillance, observation, or expectant therapy. In this option, the patient returns to his urologist every three to six months for a DRE and PSA level. If the cancer appears to be progressing, as suggested by 1) a change in symptoms, such as outlet obstructive symptoms (see Chapter 20), new onset of bone pain, or other symptoms of metastatic disease, 2) a worsening DRE, or 3) a rapid rise in the PSA level, then other treatment options can be pursued.

The best candidates for watchful waiting include:

- Men whose life expectancy is less than ten years due to age (for instance, men over 75 years old), or to illness.
- Men over the age of 70 with a well-differentiated cancer (i.e., Gleason score of 2 to 4).
- Men whose prostate cancer has spread outside the prostate but who do not have any symptoms from their cancer.
- Men who want some time to think about their options before deciding on which treatment they wish to receive.

Although watchful waiting avoids the side effects and complications associated with the other treatments for prostate cancer, it allows the cancer to grow and possibly spread. Among men with clinically localized prostate cancer and a Gleason score of 2 to 4, the cancer can be expected to spread outside the prostate in approximately 2 percent of these patients within the first year of watchful waiting, and the number increases by about 2 percent each additional year. Among similar men with a Gleason score of 7 to 10, about 14 percent develop advanced cancer during the first year of watchful waiting, and the number increases by 14 percent with each additional year. Therefore, some studies suggest that watchful waiting is an adequate option for older men with low grade cancers (Gleason score of 2 to 4). In men with moderately differentiated (Gleason score of 5 to 7) or poorly differentiated (Gleason score of 8 to 10) prostate cancer, other treatment options should be considered.

TREATMENT BY STAGE

Few absolute correct answers exist for the treatment of prostate cancer at any stage. The problems of who to treat, how to treat them, and when to treat them have not been clearly resolved by any study to date. Physicians, especially urologists, take the information that has been published about prostate cancer and try to make some sense out of it in order to form guidelines that can be used to make treatment recommendations for their patients. The treatment of prostate cancer is not as simple as making a cake by using a cookbook. Every patient and every situation is unique. The information provided in this section is based on interpretations of the current literature, and is designed to serve as a guide of the various options generally offered for the treatment of prostate cancer based on the clinical stage of the disease. It is in no way meant to be taken as "urologic law." The final decision regarding which treatment option to pursue will ultimately be based on many factors including the clinical stage and grade of the tumor, the patient's age and general health, and the patient's desires for treatment after he has received counseling from his urologist, and possibly even a second opinion.

Table 21-5: Estimated Death Rates from Untreated Prostate Cancer	
A1	2% within 5-10 years
A2	15% within 5-10 years
B1	15% within 5-10 years
B2	15-70% within 5-10 years
C	75% within 5-10 years
D1	>50% within 3 years
D2	80% within 5 years; 90% within 10 years

From: Macfarlane MT, *Urology for the House Officer, 2nd ed.* Williams and Wilkins, 1995.

A1: Only 8 to 10 percent of these cancers are expected to progress over five to eight years, and, as seen in Table 21-5, only 2 percent of these patients are expected to die of their prostate cancer within five to ten years. If the patient is likely to live ten years more or longer (for instance, if he is under age 70 and in good general health), some investigators have recommended definitive therapy with radical prostatectomy. A more conservative approach that has been recommended in these young, healthy patients with stage A1 disease is to either repeat a PSA level in three months or perform a TRUS biopsy of the prostate. If the PSA level is abnormally elevated, or if the TRUS biopsies show residual cancer, then definitive therapy is recommended. There are no data to refute the possibility that radiation therapy might be as effective as radical prostatectomy in this stage. If the PSA level is within normal limits, or if the biopsies reveal no residual cancer, follow-up DRE and PSA levels are performed every six to twelve months. In patients older than 70 years of age, or in younger patients with a less than ten-year life expectancy due to medical illness, watchful waiting is usually recommended, unless the PSA level starts to rise or the patient develops symptoms from his prostate cancer, at which point, either radiation or hormone therapy can be instituted.

A2: These patients are at much higher risk from their tumor with a 35 to 50 percent progression rate over five to eight years and 15 percent of these patients expected to die of their cancer within five to ten years if left untreated. Either radical prostatectomy or radiation therapy is generally indicated in this group, based on the age and overall health of the patient. Definitive therapy is usually delayed 6 to 12 weeks following a TURP. Radiation seed implantation may be difficult due to the paucity of prostate tissue after a TURP. Cryotherapy remains an experimental option.

Ax (B0, also known as T1c): Since in approximately 40 to 45 percent of patients being diagnosed with prostate cancer today, the only abnormality leading to the suspicion of prostate cancer is an elevated PSA level, this stage of clinical disease comprises a significant number of patients. These cancers tend to behave like A2 or B1 tumors, and therefore, patients with this stage of prostate cancer are usually offered the same treatment options as those patients with stage B1 disease.

B1: Radical prostatectomy appears to offer the best chance for cure in patients with a greater than ten year life expectancy, since 90 percent of these patients will have their cancer confined to the prostate. Fifteen-year tumor-free survivals of 50 to 75 percent have been reported following surgery. Fifteen-year survival results for external beam radiation therapy have been reported to be between 40 to 60 percent. Overall, there is no more than a 5 to 10 percent difference in the survival rates between radical prostatectomy and external beam radiation therapy, with the 15-year data slightly favoring surgery. For patients who are poor surgical risks, or for those whose life expectancy is less than ten years due to age or medical illness, radiation therapy or watchful waiting are viable options. Again, cryotherapy remains an experimental alternative.

B2: Despite all of the radiologic staging modalities presently available, 40 to 50 percent of patients with clinical stage B2 disease will be found to have cancer outside their prostate at radical prostatectomy. In spite of these staging limitations, radical prostatectomy is still recommended in young, healthy patients expected to live longer than ten years more. What to do with patients found to have cancer at the margins of the specimen (i.e., if residual tumor was probably left behind) is controversial and may depend on how much tumor is believed to have been left behind. However, if the Gleason score is less than 8, studies suggest that the patient may be followed closely (every three to six months) unless the PSA level starts to rise or the DRE becomes abnormal, at which point external radiation therapy can be instituted. In patients with both positive margins and poorly differentiated cancers (Gleason score of 8 or higher), adjuvant external radiation is usually recommended and should be delayed for a few weeks after surgery to allow ample time for healing.

For patients who do not want surgery, or for those who aren't good surgical candidates due to age or other medical illnesses, radiation therapy (either external beam or seed implants) is a viable option. In patients 75 years of age or older, watchful waiting is also an option. Cryotherapy is an experimental option for this group as well.

C: The large variety of treatments available for stage C disease suggests that no particular treatment is of major curative benefit. Presently, either radiation therapy (external beam or interstitial seeds) or hormone therapy are appropriate for patients with this stage of prostate cancer. Again, cryotherapy is an experimental option, but requires further study. Some studies have suggested that radical prostatectomy may be considered if there is low volume of disease and the Gleason score is less than 7; however, this also remains an experimental option with further study required before it can be generally recommended. Given the survival statistics for untreated stage C disease, watchful waiting does not appear to be a viable option for these patients.

D0: In the past, an elevated PAP usually indicated metastatic disease and reports have suggested that two-thirds of these patients will be found to have prostate cancer in pelvic lymph nodes at PLND; however, the false positive rate of the PAP test is approximately 7 to 20 percent. Therefore, if curative therapy is planned, pelvic lymph node dissection should be carried out, and further treatment decisions can be made based on the results of that operation. On the other hand, some investigators believe that these patients behave as though they had metastatic disease and, therefore, offer them hormone therapy.

D1: Hormone therapy is generally recommended in this group, since most investigators feel that removing the prostate, or treating it with radiation therapy, offers no survival advantage once the cancer has spread outside the prostate. The issue of when to begin hormone therapy is controversial, and no clear answer exists. Early hormone therapy involves the initiation of hormone treatment shortly after the diagnosis is made, whereas in delayed hormone therapy, treatment is not initiated unless the patient develops symptoms from his prostate cancer or the PSA level rises rapidly.

Some studies are evaluating the concomitant use of both hormone therapy and radiation therapy in this group. Other studies have advocated radical prostatectomy and immediate hormone therapy for control of local disease in certain select patients. The protocols involving radical prostatectomy in D1 prostate cancer are experimental and require further study before general recommendations other than hormone therapy can be made in this stage of disease.

D2: Hormone therapy is the treatment of choice here.

*D3:*Despite an ever-increasing amount of literature, no "standard" therapy exists for hormone resistant prostate cancer. Most people suggest that patients on pan-androgen suppression who are found to have a rising PSA level first undergo a trial of antiandrogen withdrawal (where the patient is instructed to no longer take the antiandrogen that had been prescribed), since this has been shown to result in a decrease in the PSA level in a small percentage of patients for a short period of time. Once hormone therapy is no longer effective, however, the average survival of these patients is less than one year, with 50 percent of patients surviving six months. Chemotherapy or other experimental protocols are options for these patients, but as yet, none have shown consistent appreciable responses.

Some patients can develop severe bone pain from prostate cancer which has metastasized to their bones, and this pain may be palliated with external-beam radiation aimed at these sites.

Vaccine Research

Human studies are currently in progress at a few university medical centers involving the development of a vaccine for the treatment of advanced prostate cancer. Prostate cancer cells are isolated and modified so that when injected back into the patient with advanced prostate cancer, this vaccine will stimulate the patient's immune system to fight his prostate cancer. Initial studies in rats with advanced prostate cancer showed a 30 percent long-term response. This treatment option is still at the experimental level and will require much more time and study.

CHEMOPREVENTION

Chemoprevention is the use of chemicals, either natural or synthetic, to try to prevent the development of a cancer. The Prostate Cancer Prevention Trial, a ten-year study which began in 1993, is evaluating 18,000 men older than 55 years of age and without prostate cancer. These men were divided into two groups: 1) those receiving finasteride, trade name Proscar (see Chapter 20); and 2) those receiving a placebo. The purpose of this study is to determine if Proscar, which is known to shrink the prostate, can prevent prostate cancer. Other compounds have been proposed as possible chemo-preventive agents in prostate cancer, for instance, fenretinide, a vitamin A analogue. However, these studies require many patients, a lot of money, and many years to determine the efficacy of these various compounds.

Volumes continue to be written about prostate cancer. Even though this is one of the longest chapters in this book, it scratches only the surface of this subject and presents a general overview of some of the more important points of this disease. In doing so, I wanted to give the reader a base of information upon which he or she can build. Hopefully, this chapter may help patients with prostate cancer make more informed decisions regarding their treatment. For more in-depth information on prostate cancer, I would highly recommend either of these two books:

- *The ABC's of Prostate Cancer,* by JE Oesterling and MA Moyad. Lanham, MD: Madison Books, 1997.

- *The Prostate: A Guide for Men and the Women Who Love Them,* by Walsh PC and Worthington JF. Baltimore, MD: The Johns Hopkins University Press, 1995.

Although prostate cancer is very common, most men die with prostate cancer rather than from prostate cancer. Therefore, prostate cancer is a gray-area when it comes to treatment. There is no one best treatment for everyone. Instead, patient education is crucial. Urologists, and other physicians involved, should try to give their patients as much information about their disease as possible. After discussing the different options available, we may also give our recommendations for treatment (biased though they may be). Finally, we try to help the patient arrive at the best treatment decision possible for that individual. It is still a challenge to consistently predict in which men the cancer will become clinically significant and which treatment is best for which patient. For right now, that answer is to be found somewhere in the future.

References

1. Baker LH, et al. "NCCN Prostate Cancer Practice Guidelines." *Oncology (Huntingt)* 1996; 10(11 suppl):265-288.

2. Das S and Crawford ED: *Cancer of the Prostate*. New York: Marcel Dekker, 1993.

3. Gillenwater JY, Grayhack JT, Howards SS, and Duckett JW (eds.): *Adult and Pediatric Urology*, 3rd ed. St. Louis: Mosby, 1996.

4. Hudson MA: "Screening for Prostate Cancer." *AUA Update Series* 1996; vol. 15, lesson 25.

5. Keetch DW, Andriole GL, and Catalona WJ: "Complications of Radical Retropubic Prostatectomy." *AUA Update Series* 1994; vol. 13, lesson 6.

6. Macfarlane MT: *Urology for the House Officer*, 2nd ed. Baltimore: Williams and Wilkins, 1995.

7. Nelson PS and Brawer MK: "Chemoprevention of Prostate Carcinoma." *Urology International* 1997; 4(4):7-9.

8. O'Dowd GJ, et al.: "Update on the Appropriate Staging Evaluation for Newly Diagnosed Prostate Cancer." *J Urol* 1997; 158(9):687-698

9. Oesterling JE and Moyad MA: *The ABC's of Prostate Cancer*. Lanham: Madison Books, 1997.

10. Pannek J and Partin AW: "Prostate-Specific Antigen: What's New in 1997." *Oncology* (Huntingt) 1997; 11(9):1273-1282.

11. Pisters LL and von Eschenbach AC: "Technique, Results, and Complications of 'Modern' Prostate Cryotherapy." *AUA Update Series* 1996; vol. 15, lesson 37.

12. Perrotti M and Fair WR: "Prostate Cancer Staging in the Newly Diagnosed Patient." *AUA Update Series* 1997; vol. 16, lesson 30.

13. "Prostate Cancer Awareness Week." *Ca Cancer J Clin* 1997; 47(5): 288-296.

14. Stamey TA, Ferrari MK, and Schmid HP: "The Value of Serial Prostate Specific Antigen Determinations 5 Years After Radiotherapy: Steeply Increasing Values Characterize 80 percent of Patients." *J Urol* 1993; 150(6):1856-1859.

15. Wolf JS, Jr. and Andriole GL: "The Selection of Patients for Cross-Sectional Imaging and Pelvic Lymphadenectomy Before Radical Prostatectomy." *AUA Update Series* 1997; vol. 16, lesson 15.

CHAPTER 22

BLADDER CANCER

B ladder cancer is the fourth most prevalent cancer in men and the second most common urologic malignancy, with approximately 50,000 new cases and 9,500 deaths reported in the United States each year. Since both males and females have a bladder, this is not exclusively a disease of men; however, it is seen more commonly in males than in females, with a ratio of 3:1. This chapter addresses some of the more important points regarding the diagnosis and treatment of bladder cancer. Since many of the diagnostic tests employed in the evaluation of hematuria are also used in the work-up of bladder cancer, in order to avoid repetition, I would recommend reading Chapter 18 before proceeding any further.

The bladder is basically a hollow group of muscles which stores the urine filtered by the kidneys and delivered to it by the ureters, until it is full. It then empties by muscular contractions when a person urinates. As can be seen in Figure 22-1, the bladder has four different layers:

1. *Epithelium (or urothelium):* This is the inner lining of the bladder, also known as the mucosa, which is 3 to 8 cell layers thick. The cells that make up the mucosal layer are called transitional cells, and these are the cells that can become abnormal and develop into bladder cancer.

2. *Lamina propria:* This is the spongy layer of tissue beneath the urothelium.

3. M*uscularis propria:* This is the true muscle layer of the bladder, also known as the detrusor muscle, which is divided into a superficial and deep part.

4. *Serosa:* This is the outermost layer which is surrounded by fat.

Due to various factors which will be discussed, the transitional cells that line the bladder can change their microscopic appearance. In dysplasia, the cells aren't totally normal, but they aren't definitely cancerous. Dys-

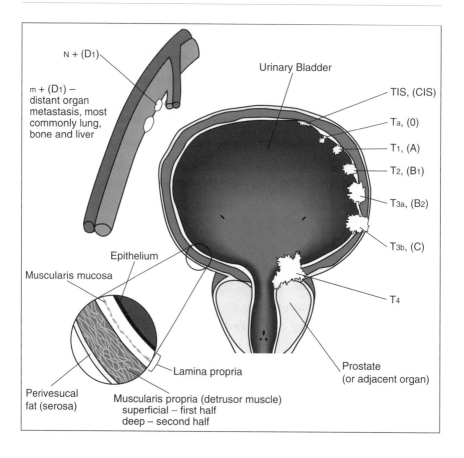

Figure 22-1: Staging of Bladder Cancer. From: Lamm DL, Torti FM: Bladder Cancer, 1996." *CA: Cancer J Clin* 1996; 26(2) 93-112. For ©American Cancer Society.

plasia is usually classified as mild, moderate, or severe, depending on how abnormal the cells are, and it can herald the development of bladder cancer. When the transitional cells of the urothelium become cancerous, the tumor that results is called transitional cell carcinoma (TCC). Carcinoma-in-situ (CIS) is defined as poorly differentiated transitional cell carcinoma that is confined to the urothelial layer. Some investigators feel that the finding of severe dysplasia in a biopsy specimen is equivalent to CIS, since it may be very difficult to distinguish the two entities. There are other types of benign and malignant tumors that can develop in the bladder; however, since 85 to 90 percent of all bladder tumors are transitional cell carcinomas, the rest of this chapter will deal specifically with transitional cell carcinoma.

Although the exact cause of bladder cancer is not known, TCC is believed to result from a combination of environmental exposure and genetic predisposition. Some of the factors that may increase a person's chances of developing bladder cancer include:

1. Cigarette smoking: It is believed that 25 to 60 percent of all cases of bladder cancer in the United States are the result of tobacco smoking. Smoking increases a person's risk of developing TCC by two to five times as compared to the general population, and although cessation of smoking can decrease a person's risk by 30 to 60 percent, it never decreases that person's risk to the level of non-smokers. It should also be noted that patients with bladder cancer who continue to smoke have been found to have an increased risk of developing other smoke-related cancers (e.g., lung cancer), in addition to recurrent bladder tumors, which is another reason for these patients to stop smoking.

2. Occupational chemical exposure: Bladder cancer was the first cancer to be identified with industrialization. Since 1895, this cancer has been associated with exposure to certain chemicals used in the dye industry (e.g., aromatic amines). Chemical workers, rubber workers, leather workers, painters, dry cleaners, and beauticians are some occupations associated with an increased risk of bladder cancer. The high risk of bladder cancer in certain occupations has led to screening studies in exposed workers at risk in an attempt to diagnose TCC at an early stage.

3. Radiation to the pelvis: In patients exposed to radiation in the area of the bladder, as might occur in the treatment of prostate cancer, the risk of TCC is 2 to 4 times greater than in the general population.

4. Analgesic abuse: High doses of pain medications containing phenacetin have been associated with an increased risk of bladder cancer.

5. Chemotherapeutic drugs: Cyclophosphamide, a drug used for the treatment of certain cancers, has been shown to increase a person's chance of developing bladder cancer for up to 6 to 13 years after treatment.

6. Chronic infection: Irritation from chronic bladder infections or foreign bodies, such as indwelling catheters, has been shown to increase the risk of developing bladder cancer. Viruses, such as human papilloma virus (see Chapter 14), have been suggested as possible causative agents

in some patients with bladder cancer, but most studies have not confirmed any role of HPV in the development of TCC of the bladder.

The role of diet in bladder cancer is controversial. Initially, caffeine was suggested to be a possible cause of bladder cancer since there appeared to be an increased association between coffee drinkers and TCC of the bladder. Subsequently, it was felt that there was no increased risk of bladder cancer with caffeine intake, and any association between the two was probably due to the finding that most coffee drinkers at that time were smokers, too. Initial studies using the artificial sweetener, saccharine, in laboratory rats suggested an increased risk of bladder cancer with high saccharine consumption; however, most recent studies have not confirmed these earlier findings.

Some studies have reported that consumption of fruits and vegetables, especially those rich in vitamin A, may lower a person's risk of developing bladder cancer. Of note, garlic may have an effect in reducing the incidence and growth of superficial bladder cancer. Further studies are needed to confirm the anti-tumor effects of garlic, but in the meantime, a little garlic can't hurt —unless you're allergic to it... or you're a vampire.

DIAGNOSIS

As discussed in other chapters, the diagnosis of any disease process is based on the history obtained from the patient, the physical examination, and certain laboratory and special studies. The diagnosis of bladder cancer is no different.

History

Bladder cancer tends to be a disease of adults, with 80 percent of these cases occurring in patients over 50 years of age. The most common symptom of bladder cancer is hematuria, either microscopic or gross, which can be intermittent. Irritative voiding symptoms (i.e., frequency, urgency, and dysuria or burning on urination) can also occur with TCC, and 30 percent of patients with a bladder cancer will have irritative voiding symptoms without hematuria. Patients with local or distant spread of their cancer may complain of weight loss, malaise, abdominal or flank pain, bone pain, leg swelling due to obstruction of lymph nodes by tumor, or symptoms of kidney problems as a result of ureteral obstruction by tumor. Since many of these symptoms can result from diseases other than bladder cancer, any person with similar symptoms should see their physician for further evaluation as soon as possible.

Physical Examination

The physical examination is usually unremarkable except in advanced disease. A bimanual examination may reveal a palpable tumor mass if the cancer is large or advanced. This exam is usually carried out at the time of cystoscopy in the office or in the operating room under anesthesia at the time of initial resection of the bladder tumor. While the patient lies on his back with his legs up in stirrups, the physician places his gloved, lubricated index finger gently into the patient's anus and advances it up into the rectum a few inches while his other hand pushes down on the lower abdomen feeling for a mass.

Laboratory Studies

Urinalysis and Urine Culture

Examination of the urine is essential to search for hematuria or evidence of infection. Hematuria requires further evaluation as discussed in Chapter 18. Since most men do not normally get urinary tract infections, the finding of a urinary tract infection may lead to further evaluation, especially in high risk individuals (e.g., smokers or those with a history of occupational or radiation exposure). It should be noted that since 30 percent of patients with bladder cancer have irritative voiding symptoms without hematuria, in patients with persistent frequency, urgency, and dysuria despite an unremarkable urinalysis and culture, further work-up is indicated to rule out a possible bladder tumor or other pathology.

Serum Creatinine

Presently, there is no blood test that can be used to screen for bladder cancer. However, before proceeding with any dye or x-ray studies, a physician may draw some blood to evaluate the patient's kidney function.

Creatinine is a chemical found in the bloodstream that is removed from the body by the kidneys. As kidney function declines, creatinine accumulates in the blood, so the higher the creatinine level, the poorer the patient's renal function. A normal creatinine level is usually less than 1.5 mg/dL, and values higher than this can increase the risk of further kidney damage with x-ray dye administration.

Special Studies

Some of the studies that may be recommended to evaluate patients suspected of having a bladder tumor include:

Intravenous Pyelogram (IVP)

This is an x-ray study that uses dye to evaluate the kidneys and ureters. It is recommended in all patients with symptoms or signs suggestive of a bladder tumor, and it is also used in patients with a known bladder tumor to rule out similar tumors in the ureters or inner lining of the kidney, which is a rare but reported occurrence in approximately 1 to 5 percent of patients with TCC of the bladder (see Chapter 18 for more details of IVP).

Cystoscopy

Under local anesthesia, a telescopic instrument is passed up the urethra and into the bladder allowing visual examination of these structures. With the advent of modern, flexible, high-quality cystoscopes, this procedure is usually performed safely in the office with minimal patient discomfort. A bladder tumor, which tends to look like a raspberry or a sea anemone (an appearance that physicians describe as papillary), will usually require further treatment in the operating room under anesthesia. Small, suspicious lesions can sometimes be biopsied in the office, but some urologists may prefer to perform biopsies under anesthesia on an outpatient basis (cystoscopy is discussed in more detail in Chapter 18).

Cytology

Cytology involves the microscopic examination of bladder (urothelial) cells by a pathologist. In this technique, fluid placed into the bladder during cystoscopy is drained from the bladder and sent to the laboratory to search for cancerous bladder cells. Cytology can be performed on voided urine, but some studies suggest that irrigating the bladder and aspirating out the fluid at the time of cystoscopy, a procedure called bladder washing, may be more accurate than cytological evaluation of voided urine alone. The problem with cytology is that the pathologist is looking at a few cells and trying to make a diagnosis. If the cells are really abnormal, as occurs in the presence of CIS, this can be an easy task. However, the cells examined may look "normal" despite the presence of a transitional cell carcinoma of the bladder. As a result, there is a false negative rate for cytology of up to 30 percent. Like many things in medicine, cytology may be helpful, but you can't rely completely on just one test. Cytology is also very helpful in the follow-up of patients with a history of bladder cancer.

Flow Cytometry

In this technique, cellular material obtained from bladder washings or tissue biopsy is processed, and a special machine is used to determine the amount of genetic material (DNA) in the urothelial cells. Cell populations with more than the normal amount of DNA have been associated with the presence of malignant transitional cell tumors in 80 percent of the cases. In addition, greater amounts of DNA in tumor cells have been associated with more aggressive cancers and a poorer prognosis.

Urinary Tumor Markers

Studies have been done to try to find proteins in the urine that are specific to bladder cancer patients (for example, bladder tumor antigen (BTA) or nuclear matrix protein (NMP 22)). The ultimate goal is to someday find a test so sensitive that you could tell whether or not a person had a bladder tumor by just examining his urine and thus, avoid routine cystoscopy. Although some of these tests have been shown to be more sensitive than cytology in the same urine specimens, at this time, cystoscopy remains the gold standard, and a tissue specimen is necessary to establish the diagnosis of bladder cancer.

Transurethral Resection of Bladder Tumor (TURBT)

If a bladder tumor is visualized, or suspected, during cystoscopy, the patient will probably be advised to undergo transurethral resection (TUR) of the lesion(s) in the operating room for both initial treatment and a definite diagnosis.

With the patient under general or spinal anesthesia, the urologist re-examines the urethra and bladder with a cystoscope. After all tumors and suspicious areas have been noted, the cystoscope is removed, and a larger cystoscopic instrument, called a resectoscope, is placed via the urethra into the bladder. The resectoscope has a wire loop which can be extended and retracted and which, when electrified, can cut through, or scrape, tissue under visual guidance. The resectoscope is used to scrape out the bladder tumors. Once the tumor(s) is resected, it is sent to the pathologist for further examination. In order to ensure that all of the tumor was resected (and to help stage the patient's cancer), a biopsy, or scraping, is taken from the base of the tumor, including some of the underlying muscle. Any abnormal-appearing areas may be biopsied to rule out CIS. Since the urothelial cells lining the bladder also line the urethra in the area of the prostate, a biopsy of the prostatic urethra is usually obtained in these patients as well. Areas of bleeding are fulgarated with the electrified loop. A urethral catheter is placed for urinary drainage. A bimanual examination is usually performed under anesthesia to search for any masses which might suggest spread of the disease.

The operation takes about 30 to 60 minutes, depending on the number and size of the bladder tumor(s). Most bladder tumors can be resected in one session; however, large tumors may require additional TURs for complete excision. The patient is usually sent home on the day of surgery, or the following morning, with antibiotics and pain medication as needed. His catheter is removed when the urine is clear, usually in one to two days. The patient is usually instructed to not take any aspirin products and to refrain from strenuous activity for one to two weeks after his surgery in an attempt to avoid hematuria.

Some of the risks of TURBT include:

1. Infection.

2. Bleeding: Although the need for transfusion after TURBT is rare, patients are advised to stop any aspirin products, or other blood thinners, at least one week before and for one to two weeks after their surgery (if their overall medical condition permits), in order to decrease the risk of bleeding during and after the operation.

3. Bladder perforation: The bladder wall is only about 1/4 of an inch thick, so attempting to scrape out a tumor, and to remove a piece of the bladder muscle with it, can result in a hole being made in the bladder. Most of the time, prolonged catheter drainage until healing occurs, usually after seven to ten days, is all that is necessary, but some perforations may require open surgery to repair.

4. Urethral stricture (i.e., narrowing of the urethra due to scarring).

5. Residual or recurrent tumors: Biopsies are usually taken at the base of the tumor site to assure that all of the tumor has been resected; however, bladder cancers can recur.

6. Catheter irritation: After TURBT, the bladder is very sensitive, and the patient feels the urge to urinate frequently until complete healing occurs. In addition, a urinary catheter can exacerbate any irritation and may result in bladder spasms which are perceived as crampy pains in the lower abdomen and which usually resolve once the catheter is removed. Medications may also be prescribed to try to relax the bladder muscle and make the catheter more "tolerable."

7. Irritative voiding symptoms: Frequency, urgency, and dysuria can persist for a few weeks after TURBT until the raw areas in the bladder heal, but the urologist can prescribe certain medications that may diminish the severity of these symptoms.

8. Anesthetic risks (i.e., heart attack and death) which, although present, are rare.

After the TURBT has been performed, the tissue obtained is sent to the pathologist for examination. Once the presence of transitional cell carcinoma is confirmed, two important factors that need to be considered before further treatment recommendations can be considered are the grade and stage of the patient's cancer.

GRADE

When describing the cancer found in the TUR specimen, the pathologist will usually assign a grade to the tumor. Grade refers to the degree of differentiation of the cancer cells, or how closely they resemble normal bladder cells. In grading, the microscopic appearance of the tumor cells is used to predict how aggressive, or fast-growing, they are. That is, the more the tumor cells look like normal bladder urothelium, the less aggressive the tumor is likely to be, and the better the patient's prognosis. TCC of the bladder is graded as:

Grade 1

- Well-differentiated (i.e., the tumor cells closely resemble normal bladder cells).

Grade 2

- Moderately differentiated (i.e., more profound abnormalities than those seen in grade 1 tumors). These tumors tend to have variable degrees of aggressiveness.

Grade 3

- Poorly differentiated (i.e., very profound abnormalities in the cancer cells). Sometimes, the abnormalities may be so severe that it can be difficult to tell that these are bladder cancer cells without knowing where the specimen came from. These are very aggressive cancers, and 50 percent of grade 3 transitional cell carcinomas are muscle-invasive at the time of diagnosis.

STAGE

Stage refers to the depth of invasion, or, in other words, how far the tumor has spread into the surrounding tissues or to other parts of the body, if at all. It is the single most important prognostic factor for the patient with

TCC of the bladder. The two staging systems in common use today are the ABCD system, also known as the Jewett-Marshall system, and the more recent international TNM classification, which stands for T - tumor, N - nodes (i.e., lymph node involvement), and M - metastases (i.e., distant spread of cancer).

In the Jewett-Marshall system:

- **Stage 0** is defined as a superficial papillary tumor confined to the mucosa with no invasion, or carcinoma in situ (CIS).

- **Stage A** is a papillary tumor invading the lamina propria.

- **Stage B1** describes a tumor extending into the superficial part of the detrusor muscle (i.e., minimal muscle invasion).

- **Stage B2** refers to tumor that extends into the deep part of the bladder muscle layer.

- **Stage C** describes a tumor that extends through the entire thickness of the bladder wall and invades the fat around the bladder, also called the perivesical fat.

- **Stage D1** occurs when the TCC involves adjacent structures, such as the prostate, or spreads to the lymph nodes around the bladder.

- **Stage D2** refers to tumor that has spread to distant organs, such as liver, lung, or bone.

In the TNM classification, three aspects of the cancer are usually specified: T describes the tumor, N describes any lymph node involvement, and M refers to the presence of metastatic spread of disease:

- **T0** implies no evidence of tumor.

- **Tis** refers to carcinoma in situ.

- **Ta** describes a papillary tumor confined to the mucosa (i.e., non-invasive).

- **T1** is used to signify tumor that invades the lamina propria.

- **T2** refers to cancer extending into the superficial layer of bladder muscle.

- **T3a** describes cancer invading the deep muscle layer.

- **T3b** occurs when the tumor spreads outside the bladder to involve the perivesical fat.

- **T4** describes tumor invading adjacent structures, such as the prostate.

- **N0** signifies that no lymph nodes near the bladder have been invaded by cancer.

- **N1** denotes that cancer has spread to one lymph node (smaller than 2 cm).

- **N2** occurs when the cancer has spread to one lymph node and caused it to become 2-5 cm in size, or to multiple lymph nodes, all totaling less than 5 cm in size.

- **N3** signifies that cancer in the lymph nodes has achieved a size of 5 cm or larger.

- **M0** signifies no evidence of distant cancer spread.

- **M1** indicates that the cancer has spread far beyond the bladder (e.g., to the liver, lungs, or bones).

A comparison of the two staging systems is seen in Table 22-1.

Table 22-1: Summary of the TNM and Jewett-Marshall Staging Systems		
TNM	**JM**	**What the Results Mean**
T0	-	No cancer.
Tis	0	CIS
Ta	0	Papillary TCC confined to the mucosa, no invasion.
T1	A	Lamina propia invasion.
T2	B1	Invasion of the superficial part of the muscle layer.
T3a	B2	Deep muscle invasion.
T3b	C	Extension to the perivesical fat.
T4	D1	Invasion of adjacent pelvic organs (e.g., prostate).
N0	-	No lymph nodes have been invaded by cancer.
N1-3	D1	Spread to pelvic lymph nodes around the bladder.
M0	-	No distant metastases.
M1	D2	The cancer has spread far beyond the bladder (e.g., to the liver, lungs, or bones).

Superficial bladder cancer is a term used to describe TCC confined to the mucosa or lamina propria (i.e., Ta, Tis, or T1). Superficial bladder cancers usually require no further staging evaluations; however, in patients with muscle-invasive TCC, or those suspected of having disease outside the bladder, additional tests may be recommended to help estimate the stage of the patient's cancer and to guide treatment recommendations. Some staging studies that may be used include:

1. *Chest X-ray (CXR):* This is a good initial study to search for tumor spread to the lungs. Any suspicious lesions will require further evaluation, possibly with a CT scan of the chest.

2. *Computed axial tomography scan (CT scan):* This is an x-ray study during which the patient lies on a table that is passed through a circular machine that looks like a big donut. With the help of a computer, this x-ray machine makes cross-sectional images of the body. It is used to search for enlarged lymph nodes around the bladder, or to find evidence of metastatic disease. Since an iodine-based contrast solution is administered intravenously to help visualize certain structures, the risks of CT scan are similar to those for IVP (see Chapter 18). Unfortunately, cancer spreads outside the bladder on a microscopic level first before causing visually-appreciable changes in the lymph nodes or other organs; therefore, the false-negative rate of CT scan (i.e., the possibility that the scan will appear normal even in the presence of disease outside the bladder) is approximately 40 percent. CT scan primarily serves a role in staging large or bulky bladder tumors and as a baseline to assess responses to radiation or chemotherapy.

3. *Magnetic Resonance Imaging (MRI):* This study uses magnetic waves, instead of x-rays, to take pictures of the patient's internal organs. The patient is required to lie still for 30 to 40 minutes in a small tube-shaped chamber while the films are obtained. The overall accuracy of MRI in the staging of bladder cancer is similar to CT scan, although some studies report that MRI is slightly better than CT scan at staging bladder cancer. Some drawbacks of MRI include: 1) patients who are claustrophobic may not be able to tolerate the small space for the time required to complete the study, and 2) patients with pacemakers and other metallic implants may not be able to be scanned.

4. *Bone Scan:* This is a diagnostic test used to search for the spread of TCC to a patient's bones. In this study, a radioactive solution is injected

intravenously. The nuclear material, or tracer as it is also known, accumulates in areas of bone that are trying to regenerate. Areas of bone to which bladder cancer has spread will concentrate the nuclear tracer, and this will show up on a machine that detects radioactivity. Other conditions may cause tracer to accumulate in bones and thus may cause a false positive scan. Some of these include: arthritis, old fractures, or infections in the bone. Bone scans are only recommended for patients with skeletal symptoms (new onset of bone pain) or an elevated alkaline phosphatase. The latter is a chemical in the blood that, when elevated, may be a sign of tumor spread to bone.

Once the clinical stage of the patient's bladder cancer is estimated, the urologist usually reviews all of the information with the patient, discusses the various treatment options available, and makes recommendations for the further treatment of the patient's TCC. These recommendations are based on many pieces of information, including the general health of the patient, and the grade and estimated stage of the patient's cancer. Although treatment preferences and recommendations may vary, treatment options are usually based on whether the bladder cancer is 1) superficial (i.e., Ta, T1, or Tis); 2) muscle-invasive (i.e., T2 or T3a); or 3) advanced or metastatic (i.e., T3b, T4, N+, or M+). The next section will discuss the more commonly recommended treatment options for each of the various stages of TCC of the bladder.

SUPERFICIAL TCC

The initial management of superficial transitional cell carcinoma of the bladder involves TURBT. Some urologists use laser to burn or vaporize bladder tumors. This procedure is performed in a manner similar to TURBT, but instead of using an electrified loop to scrape out the tumor, a laser is used to destroy it. Some advantages of the laser include minimal blood loss and less risk of perforation. A disadvantage is that no tissue can be obtained with the laser. Therefore, in patients treated with laser, biopsies of the tumor are usually obtained first to be able to evaluate it pathologically. Then, the laser is used to destroy the cancer. Most urologists today still use the resectoscope and electrified loop to perform TURBT to treat TCC of the bladder and to obtain specimen for the pathologist to examine.

Stage Ta (Stage 0)

TURBT is curative in most of these cases with five-year survival rates reported to be at least 95 percent. In those tumors found to be low grade (grade 1), only TURBT and close follow-up are usually recommended. Since approximately 50 percent of these cancers will recur, even up to many years after the initial diagnosis, lifelong surveillance is recommended. The traditional follow-up for patients with superficial TCC involves serial cystoscopy and bladder washing for cytology every three months for two years, then every six months for the next two years, and annually thereafter. Also, due to the slight increased risk of development of similar cancers in the ureters or lining of the kidneys, a yearly IVP has also been recommended in those patients with normal renal function. If, however, the tumor is high grade (grade 2 to 3), larger than 5 cm, or found in multiple sites in the bladder, or if the patient is found to have a rapid recurrence of TCC on his three month follow-up cystoscopy, additional intravesical therapy may be recommended to try to decrease the risk of future recurrences (see the section on intravesical therapy, page 228).

Stage T1 (Stage A)

This stage of disease tends to be very aggressive with many of these lesions being high grade (i.e., grade 2 or 3) and recurrence rates of 75 percent with 25 to 30 percent of these recurrences progressing to muscle-invasive disease. Therefore, in patients with T1 TCC, treatment with TURBT alone is not sufficient, and additional intravesical therapy is usually recommended (see the section on intravesical therapy). Five-year survival rates with TURBT and intravesical therapy have been reported to be approximately 72 percent. Failure to respond to intravesical therapy is usually an indication for surgical removal of the bladder (i.e., radical cystectomy). Routine follow-up of T1 TCC is as described for stage Ta.

Carcinoma-in-situ (Tis or CIS)

Despite its superficial location, this stage of disease is very aggressive. Treatment with TURBT and fulgaration alone tends to result in recurrence rates of 70 to 82 percent, with 50 to 80 percent progressing to more advanced disease, and only a 60 percent five-year survival rate. Therefore, TURBT alone is not definitive treatment for most patients with CIS. Years ago, the treatment of choice for CIS was radical cystectomy; however, now intravesical therapy (see below), which has had excellent results in decreasing the recurrence rates of CIS, is usually recommended as first line therapy for CIS following TURBT. Failure to respond to intravesical therapy is an indication for radical cystectomy. Routine follow-up of CIS is as described for stage Ta.

Intravesical Therapy

Intravesical therapy was designed in an attempt to decrease recurrences of TCC and, hopefully, to delay or prevent the need for radical cystectomy. It basically consists of various medications which are instilled into the bladder via a catheter. The patient is asked to retain the solution in the bladder for a certain period of time, after which he urinates it out. The commonly accepted indications for intravesical therapy after TURBT include: 1) the presence of CIS; 2) lamina propria invasion (T1 or stage A TCC); 3) high grade tumor; 4) multiple tumors found at TURBT; 5) large tumor size (greater than 5 cm); and 6) rapid tumor recurrence.

There are two common forms of intravesical therapy currently in use: intravesical immunotherapy, and intravesical chemotherapy (not to be confused with systemic chemotherapy which is administered intravenously and is generally used to treat metastatic TCC).

Intravesical Immunotherapy

This form of therapy is believed to stimulate the body's immune system to fight residual microscopic cancer and prevent recurrent disease. The most common agent used for intravesical immunotherapy is bacillus Calmette-Guerin (BCG) which is a mild form of the organism that causes tuberculosis. BCG has proven to be the most successful form of immunotherapy for the treatment of superficial bladder cancer to date, and as a result, is the current treatment of choice for aggressive superficial TCC (i.e., T1, Tis, and high grade Ta).

A delay in the initiation of treatment for ten or more days after TURBT is usually recommended to allow the bladder to heal and to lessen the risk of side effects. The patient comes to the office without the need for prior preparation. A urinalysis is usually performed to rule out any infection (which is a contraindication to administration of the BCG). A catheter is inserted via the urethra into the bladder, and the BCG mixture is allowed to drip into the bladder without pressure. The patient is instructed to try to retain the BCG in his bladder for as long as possible, up to 2 hours, and then, to urinate it out.

The optimal dosage and treatment schedule for BCG remains undefined, and patients may be treated with different schedules depending on their urologist's training. However, one recommended schedule calls for the patient to receive intravesical BCG once a week for six weeks, then receive an additional three weekly instillations, given three months after the initiation of treatment, and another three weekly instillations at six months after the initiation of treatment. Some investigators feel that the three additional weekly treatments repeated at six month intervals for up to three years thereafter (called maintenance BCG therapy) may help decrease recurrence rates even further, but maintenance therapy is controversial at this time. The decision to give maintenance BCG treatments might be based on patient risk factors, since it is unlikely that all patients will require it.

The follow-up of patients receiving intravesical BCG is as described for superficial TCC. It includes cystoscopy and washings for cytology every three months for the first two years, then every six months for the next two years, and annually thereafter. In addition, some researchers recommend an annual IVP.

Patients receiving BCG treatments are advised to refrain from taking aspirin products, or other anti-inflammatory medications (for example, ibuprofen), since these drugs are believed to decrease the efficacy of BCG by preventing the organism from binding to the bladder wall.

Contraindications to the administration of BCG include: immunosuppressed patients (e.g., AIDS patients or those with cancers, such as leukemia or Hodgkin's disease), pregnant or lactating females, patients with a urinary tract infection or inflamed bladders, or patients with active tuberculosis. If significant difficulty is encountered placing the catheter for BCG administration or if the patient is suspected of having a urinary tract infection, it is recommended that the treatment be delayed a few days to allow healing, and treatment of any infection, since traumatic catheterization and/or urinary tract infection can increase the risk of complications from BCG.

The vast majority of patients receiving BCG have no significant complications; however, some of the common side effects of BCG therapy include:

1. Irritative voiding symptoms (reported in 80 to 90 percent of patients): These symptoms of frequency, urgency, and dysuria usually begin after the second or third instillation and persist for about two days. For those patients with severe symptoms, certain medications can be prescribed to try to minimize discomfort.

2. Flu-like symptoms (25 percent): Malaise, low-grade fever, muscle aches, and nausea may occur, but usually resolve by one to two days after administration with Tylenol and fluids.

3. Fever over 103° F (2.9 percent): This also usually resolves in one to two days; however, high fever can also be a sign of a serious systemic BCG infection. Therefore, any patient who develops a fever of over 103° F after BCG administration is usually hospitalized for observation and treated with anti-tuberculous medication.

4. Gross hematuria (1 percent): Although microscopic hematuria is more common during these treatments, gross hematuria can occur and may be very alarming to the patient.

5. Prostatitis (0.9 percent): This results from spread of the BCG organism to the prostate. The inflammation and scarring that result from this infection can cause the prostate to develop areas of firmness which may not be distinguishable from prostate cancer without a prostate biopsy.

6. Systemic tuberculosis involving the lung or liver (0.7 percent): This requires treatment for tuberculosis and cessation of intravesical BCG administration.

7. Severe allergic reaction to BCG, called BCG sepsis (0.4 percent): This requires hospitalization, treatment with anti-tuberculous medications and steroids, and cessation of intravesical BCG administration.

8. Arthralgia, or temporary joint pains (0.5 percent).

9. Skin rash (0.3 percent).

10. Epididymo-orchitis (0.4 percent): see Chapter 15.

11. Bladder scarring (0.2 percent).

Life-threatening and fatal complications have been reported with BCG therapy, but these are exceedingly rare.

BCG has been shown to significantly reduce the chance of tumor recurrence and progression when compared to no treatment or intravesical chemotherapy, with cancer-free response rates of 70 to 82 percent. It is currently the most effective intravesical therapy available for the treatment of superficial bladder cancer.

Some of the other agents currently being evaluated for their efficacy as immunotherapeutic drugs include: 1) interferon; 2) keyhole limpet hemo-cyanin (KLH), a protein found in a marine mollusk; 3) bropirimine; 4) tumor necrosis factor; 5) interleukin-2; 6) irradiated tumor vaccine; and 7) garlic. The preliminary results with many of these agents have been promising, but further studies are needed to define and confirm their roles in the treatment of superficial TCC.

Intravesical Chemotherapy

This mode of treatment involves the instillation of anti-cancer drugs into the bladder via a catheter in an attempt to kill residual tumor cells and decrease the incidence of recurrent tumors. Various drugs have been tried (e.g., thiotepa, mitomycin C (MMC), and doxorubicin) with MMC being the most effective chemotherapeutic agent so far.

The optimal doses and treatment schedules for the various intravesical chemotherapeutic drugs also remain undefined. In general, patients receive weekly instillations for 6 to 8 weeks. Recent studies suggest that, as opposed to BCG where early instillation is contraindicated, early intravesical instil-lation of chemotherapeutic agents (i.e., within 24 hours of TURBT), may reduce tumor recurrence rates. The theory is that early instillation of these drugs may kill residual tumor cells floating in the bladder after TURBT and thus, prevent them from implanting, or attaching and growing, somewhere else in the bladder.

The follow-up of patients receiving intravesical chemotherapy is as described for patients with superficial TCC.

Like intravesical immunotherapy, these treatments also tend to be well tolerated. Some of the side effects of intravesical chemotherapy include: 1) irritative voiding symptoms (10 to 20 percent); 2) genital rash (5 percent): seen mostly with MMC, so meticulous attention to washing of the hands and genitalia after MMC instillation and the first post-treatment void is recommended; 3) low blood counts (4 percent): These are chemotherapy drugs, so absorption of these agents into the bloodstream can result in suppression of blood counts, similar to the effects seen with systemic chemotherapy. The risk of this side effect is greatest with the drug thiotepa, so blood counts are usually monitored while patients are receiving thiotepa instillations; and 4) bladder scarring, which is a rare side effect.

Most of the intravesical chemotherapeutic agents have similar efficacy in preventing cancer recurrence in patients with superficial TCC, but MMC appears to be slightly more effective than the other agents. Cancer recurrence rates are reduced to about 30 to 40 percent as compared with 70 percent in a control group treated with TURBT alone.

Due to the fact that the mechanism of action for BCG is different from that of the chemotherapeutic agents, patients who have failed to respond to intravesical chemotherapy may respond to BCG, and vice versa.

Due to the efficacy of TURBT and intravesical therapeutic management, the majority of patients with superficial TCC rarely require open surgery. Indications for radical cystectomy to manage superficial disease include persistent or recurrent high-grade tumor despite intravesical therapy, or progression to a higher stage (to muscle-invasive disease) on follow-up evaluation. Cystectomy has achieved a high cure rate for superficial TCC of the bladder. Some studies report cancer-specific five-year survival rates of 88 percent for Ta, 76 percent for T1, and close to 100 percent for CIS.

MUSCLE-INVASIVE TCC

There are various treatment options for patients with muscle-invasive TCC (i.e., T2 or T3a).

Radical Cystectomy

Radical cystectomy is the surgical removal of the bladder, prostate, seminal vesicles, and perivesical fat. It is the most common treatment for muscle-invasive bladder cancer in the United States, and remains the standard against which other forms of therapy for invasive TCC are measured.

Before surgery, a few steps are usually taken to optimize conditions for the procedure:

1. It is recommended that the patient stops using any aspirin, ibuprofen, or other blood-thinners, at least 1 week before surgery to try to prevent excessive bleeding during or after the operation.

2. Since some patients lose enough blood to require a blood transfusion during or after their surgery, in the days or weeks before radical cystectomy, the patient may be asked to donate his own blood to have it available in case he needs a transfusion during or after the operation. This technique is called autologous blood donation.

3. Since a portion of the intestines is used to form a conduit or a reservoir for urinary diversion after radical cystectomy, the intestinal tract is emptied and sterilized. On the day before the operation, patients are asked to drink preparations designed to clean out their intestines (e.g., Golytely, which makes you "go" a lot). Cleansing enemas may be used to clean out the rectum on the evening prior to surgery. Oral antibiotics are given to sterilize the intestines, and intravenous antibiotics are also administered before surgery to decrease infectious complications.

4. Because the urinary stream may need to be diverted to an opening on the abdominal wall (i.e., a stoma site), which can be covered by a collection device, or drainage bag, the optimal site for this stoma will be marked by the surgeon or a stoma nurse on the day prior to the operation. The stoma is usually located on the right side of the lower

abdomen about two inches below and two to three inches lateral to the belly-button.

5. Some urologists recommend special inflatable stockings known as sequential compression stockings, or small amounts of blood-thinning agents (e.g., heparin) to be used shortly before and immediatly post-operatively in an attempt to decrease the risk of blood clot formation in the legs or blood vessels around the bladder.

6. In an attempt to kill any cancer cells in the bladder, and thus to decrease the risk of spilling live tumor cells into the wound during the surgery, some urologists may instill a chemotherapeutic agent into the bladder (for example, thiotepa) in the operating room just before beginning the surgery.

The patient is usually admitted to the hospital on the day before the surgery, so some of the preparatory measures just described can be carried out under supervision. The operation is usually performed under general anesthesia with the patient lying flat. If removal of the entire urethra is also planned (i.e., a urethrectomy), however, then the patient's legs will be placed up in stirrups. A vertical skin incision is made in the midline from 3 cm above the belly-button to just above the penis, curving around the belly-button on the side opposite the stoma mark. The lymph nodes around the bladder are sampled first. This part of the operation is called a pelvic lymph node dissection (PLND), and is used to determine the stage of the patient's cancer further.

Some studies have reported that PLND may prolong survival in TCC patients with minimal spread of their cancer to the lymph nodes as compared to similar patients treated with radical cystectomy without PLND. However, if there appears to be a large amount of cancer in the lymph nodes around the bladder, radical cystectomy does not appear to offer any survival advantage. In this situation, rather than expose the patient to the risks of major surgery, possibly without any significant benefits, the operation is usually aborted, the patient's incision is closed, and other treatment options for advanced bladder cancer are subsequently discussed with the patient (e.g., systemic chemotherapy). On the other hand, if the disease does not appear to have spread outside the bladder, the ureters are cut away from the bladder; the bladder, prostate, and seminal vesicles are dissected free from surrounding structures; the prostate is cut away from the urethra; and then the entire specimen (bladder, prostate and seminal vesicles) is removed and sent to the pathologist for microscopic examination and final pathologic staging. Urethrectomy (i.e., removal of the urethra) may also be performed at the time of radical cystectomy if the patient was found to have TCC involving the prostatic urethra on biopsies obtained at the time of TURBT.

The nerves and blood vessels responsible for erections run along the posterior aspect of both sides of the prostate. Due to the development of the technique by Dr. Patrick Walsh of the John's Hopkins Hospital, these nerves can sometimes be dissected away from the bladder and prostate in an attempt to preserve sexual function in patient's undergoing radical cystectomy. This technique is known as the nerve-sparing approach.

Once the specimen has been removed, some form of urinary diversion procedure is performed to deal with the flow of urine from the kidneys and ureters. There are two basic forms of urinary diversions, and they are both made from a piece of the patient's own intestines: intestinal conduits, and continent reservoirs.

Intestinal Conduits

Various segments of intestines have been used to divert the urine after radical cystectomy, but the most popular form of urinary diversion with the lowest complication rate is the ileal conduit. In the ileal conduit, a piece of intestine about 6 to 10 inches long is taken from the intestinal tract. The ureters are sewn into one end of this tube, and the other end is brought out through a hole, or stoma, made in the skin of the lower abdominal wall. Urine flows from the ureters, through the piece of intestine (now called a conduit), out the stoma, and into a collection bag that covers the stoma and which is emptied by the patient when full. This sounds horrible initially, but most patients tolerate it very well. It should be noted that despite all the fears of alteration of body image with intestinal conduits, in one study, 70 percent of patients reported no change in their social activities after ileal conduit diversion, 20 percent reported less social activity, and 10 percent reported more social activity after diversion. One-third considered fear of accidental leakage of urine from the collecting device as the most negative aspect of treatment.

Continent Urinary Diversion

The ability to create a continent urinary reservoir that does not require an external appliance is one of the most important recent advances in the treatment of invasive bladder cancer. In these operations, a piece of intestine is isolated and used to make a pouch, or reservoir. The ureters are sewn into one end of the pouch. Then, if a urethrectomy was not performed, the pouch can be sewn to the remaining stump of urethra to create an artificial bladder, called a neobladder, which may allow the patient to urinate when the pouch is full. On the other hand, the pouch can be connected to a small opening in the abdominal wall in such a manner that urine will be retained in the pouch until the patient passes a catheter into the pouch to drain it every few hours, thus avoiding the need for an external drainage bag. Continent diversions require longer operating time, are technically more difficult to perform, and have a higher complication rate than the intestinal conduits.

No matter what type of urinary diversion is performed, catheters for urinary drainage are sometimes temporarily placed in the ureters until the connections between the ureters and the piece of intestines heal (usually 10 to 14 days).

Radical cystectomy usually takes about four to five hours, but can take longer if a continent diversion is performed. Patients generally have a tube placed via their nose into their stomach, called a nasogastric tube (NG tube), to drain stomach secretions until the intestines start to function again, which usually takes four to five days. After this, the NG tube is removed, and the patient's diet is slowly advanced until he's eating real food. The usual hospital stay is seven to ten days, but every patient is different. Patients are instructed in the care of their urinary diversion, and are usually proficient at this task by the time of, or shortly after, discharge. Patients are discharged home with pain medication as needed and oral antibiotics. They are advised not to drive for two weeks and to refrain from any strenuous activity or heavy lifting for four to six weeks. Walking, however, is encouraged.

After surgery, patients are usually followed-up every 3 to 6 months for a few years and then, annually with various studies including blood work and chest x-rays, and possibly a yearly CT scan, to search for evidence of recurrent tumor or metastatic disease.

Although radical cystectomy is considered the most effective treatment for patients with muscle-invasive TCC of the bladder, many people fear its associated morbidity. Some of the complications that have been reported after radical cystectomy include:

1. Infection (5 percent).

2. Bleeding requiring transfusion (3 percent): In an attempt to avoid using any blood from the blood bank, autologous blood donation has been employed. In addition, now there are machines that allow surgeons to collect blood that is lost during surgery, and after processing, this blood can be given back to the patient. However, even with all of these precautions, there is still a rare possibility that the patient may lose enough blood to require a transfusion from the blood bank. Blood is now screened for hepatitis and AIDS, so although there are still risks associated with banked blood, they are low.

3. Delayed return of intestinal function, known as prolonged ileus (6 percent).

4. Opening of the patient's incision, known as wound dehiscence (3 percent).

5. Small bowel obstruction (3 percent): When the piece of intestines to be used in urinary diversion is removed, the remaining open ends of the patient's intestines are sewn together again to reconstitute the intestinal tract for food passage. Swelling or scarring in the area of this junction can cause obstruction to the flow of food, resulting in abdominal pain, nausea, and vomiting. Also, scarring that develops in the belly cavity as a result of surgery may obstruct the bowels up to years after the operation causing similar symptoms.

6. Rectal injury (2.4 percent): A hole can be made in the rectum at the time of surgery. It is usually apparent, and suture closure of the hole is usually all that is required for repair.

7. Damage to adjacent structures, such as blood vessels.

8. Pain: This is major surgery, but post-operatively, various medications are used to keep the patient comfortable. Chronic pain, in the absence of metastatic disease, is rare.

9. Hernia (2 to 3 percent): Weaknesses can develop in the area of the incision, or around the stoma site, so patients are advised to avoid strenuous activity for four to six weeks after their surgery.

10. Deep vein thrombosis and/or pulmonary embolus: During this procedure, patients lie on the operating table for 4 or more hours while the urologist operates around blood vessels in the pelvis. As a result, clots may form in the veins that drain the blood from the legs, a condition known as deep vein thrombosis (DVT). Symptoms of DVT include asymmetric swelling, or pain, in the legs, but DVT can be present without symptoms. Occasionally, these clots can break loose and travel through the bloodstream to lodge in the lungs, a condition known as a pulmonary embolus (PE), which can be fatal. Symptoms of PE include fever, shortness of breathe, and a rapid heart rate. Some steps may be taken to try to decrease the risk of DVT or PE. These include: a) the use of compression stockings; b) the use of blood-thinners for a short time after the surgery; and c) having the patient move his legs and get up and walk as soon as possible after the operation.

11. Urine leak: Sometimes, the site where the ureters are sewn to the intestinal segment (i.e. the uretero-intestinal anastomosis) may leak urine. Temporary ureteral catheters, or stents, have been placed at the time of surgery to decrease this risk until healing occurs (usually 10 to 14 days).

12. Impotence: If the nerve-sparing procedure is not performed, the risk of impotence is approximately 100 percent. If the nerves are spared, potency rates of up to 60 percent have been reported. The best chance of preserving sexual function if the nerves are spared occurs in men less than 60 years of age. It can take up to 1 year after surgery for sexual function to return, if at all. In the meantime, and even if permanent impotence does occur, there are many successful treatment options available today to help patients improve their sex life (see Chapter 6).

13. Uretero-intestinal anastomotic stricture (5 to 10 percent): This occurs when scar tissue narrows or occludes the site where the ureter is sewn to the piece of intestine. Various surgical procedures have been designed to deal with this problem with good success rates.

14. Residual or recurrent tumor.

15. Metabolic complications: All forms of urinary diversion using intestinal segments can cause metabolic derangements, but these tend to be more pronounced in continent diversions than in conduits. With close medical follow-up, these derangements rarely lead to significant problems.

16. Kidney stones (6 to 13 percent): Intestinal conduits are associated with a higher risk of kidney stone formation than in the general population, possibly due to the increased incidence of urinary tract infections in these patients.

17. Heart attack and/or death (2 percent).

Results of various studies reveal an overall 5-year survival rate for patients undergoing radical cystectomy for invasive bladder cancer to be approximately 50 percent. Survival rates are related to the final pathologic stage of the cancer, as determined by the pathologist's microscopic examination of the specimen. In one study, five-year survival rates were 75 percent for patients with T1 disease, 63 percent for patients with T2 disease, 31 percent for patients with T3 cancer, and 21 percent for those with T4 TCC.

Adjuvant Chemotherapy

Radical cystectomy provides excellent local control of bladder cancer; however, 50 percent of all patients with muscle-invasive bladder cancer, independent of the type of treatment they receive, subsequently die of metastatic disease. It has been postulated that once bladder cancer gets into the muscle layer, microscopic spread of the cancer cells outside the bladder occurs rapidly. Therefore, many patients with muscle-invasive bladder cancer may have microscopic disease outside the bladder, which is not readily apparent at the time of radical cystectomy, and these tumor cells can become manifest as recurrent or metastatic disease at some time after the operation. As a result, it has been suggested that the intravenous admini-stration of chemotherapeutic drugs to patients with microscopic evidence of TCC outside the bladder may prolong survival by killing any possible tumor cells left behind in these patients, even if the margins of resection are free of tumor. The technique of giving additional therapy after radical surgery is called adjuvant therapy, and in this situation is known as adjuvant chemotherapy.

Studies in patients found to have locally advanced bladder cancer at the time of radical cystectomy (i.e., T3b disease) have shown that adjuvant chemotherapy delays cancer progression and prolongs survival, as com-pared to radical cystectomy alone.

M-VAC chemotherapy (the letters represent the first letter of each chemotherapeutic agent used: methotrexate, vinblastine, adriamycin, and cis-platin) has been the most effective form of adjuvant therapy so far. There is no work that has demonstrated a beneficial role for adjuvant chemother-apy in the treatment of T2 TCC.

Bladder Preservation

Some patients with muscle-invasive bladder cancer are not candidates for radical cystectomy due to poor medical health or extreme age, while other patients absolutely refuse to undergo radical surgery. Radiation therapy, chemotherapy, local resection, and various combinations of these treatment modalities have been studied in an attempt to treat invasive bladder cancer while preserving bladder function. The best candidates for "bladder-sparing" treatment are those whose tumors are relatively small, well-circumscribed, and solitary. Unfortunately, since approximately 30 to 70 percent of patients with muscle-invasive TCC can be found to have areas of CIS elsewhere in the bladder, this normally constitutes a small group of patients.

Transurethral Resection (TUR)

Transurethral resection is not considered standard therapy for muscle-invasive TCC; however, some studies have shown five-year survival rates exceeding 80 percent and bladder preservation rates of 70 percent in highly selected patients treated with TURBT. In patients with well-circumscribed, solitary, papillary tumors amenable to complete resection, TURBT has been used in experimental protocols with good results. TURBT, with or without intravesical therapy, may be an option for those patients who are medically unfit for, or who absolutely refuse, radical cystectomy and other treatment options.

Partial Cystectomy

Partial cystectomy involves removing only that portion of the bladder that has the tumor in the hope of avoiding the need for cystectomy. In this procedure, usually performed under general anesthesia, a vertical incision is made in the lower abdomen, and the bladder is exposed. The bladder is opened, and the area of tumor is excised along with a 2 cm. margin of normal-appearing tissue around the tumor itself. Since the tumor may be found to not be amenable to partial cystectomy at the time of surgery, the patient may require a radical cystectomy, but that decision may only be possible to make during the operation itself. In fact, in one study, only 6 to 19 percent of patients with muscle-invasive bladder cancer met the selection criteria for partial cystectomy; therefore, the patient is usually counseled and prepared for possible radical cystectomy.

The principal drawback of partial cystectomy is a 38 to 78 percent risk of local recurrence; however, in patients with highly localized T2 lesions, the reported five-year survival rates of 50 to 70 percent are comparable to those in contemporary series of patients treated with radical cystectomy.

Radiation Therapy

External-beam radiation therapy has been used to treat muscle-invasive bladder cancer, especially in Europe and Canada. In this form of therapy, the patient lies on a table, and a machine focuses x-ray beams on the bladder and local lymph nodes to destroy cancer cells. Each treatment session lasts 15 to 30 minutes, with the entire course of therapy usually taking four to seven weeks to complete. After this, the patient is followed closely by his urologist with frequent cystoscopy and/or biopsies as discussed in the section on superficial TCC. Follow-up blood work, chest x-rays, and CT scans may also be performed to screen for the development of advanced or metastatic disease.

Some of the risks of radiation therapy include 1) impotence; 2) gastro-intestinal problems, such as diarrhea (up to 70 percent during treatment, but only seen in 10 percent of patients long-term); and 3) urinary problems, such as hematuria and irritative voiding symptoms (10 percent long-term).

The real problem with radiation therapy is that, used alone, it is inferior to radical cystectomy. Up to 50 percent of patients with invasive TCC treated with radiation therapy will develop recurrent or persistent disease requiring salvage radical cystectomy. Unfortunately, by that time, only 8 to 15 percent of patients who are not cured by radiation will be suitable candidates for the operation. Five-year survival rates for patients with muscle-invasive disease treated with radiation therapy have been reported to be approximately 24 percent.

Combined Therapy

Various combinations of radiation therapy and chemotherapy, with or without bladder preserving surgery, have been attempted in experimental studies; however, more information is needed to determine the overall effectiveness of these "bladder-conserving" strategies for patients with muscle-invasive TCC of the bladder.

In summary, the recommended treatment of choice for patients with muscle-invasive bladder cancer is radical cystectomy with some form of urinary diversion. At this point, it appears that bladder preservation is an option for a minority of patients who absolutely refuse, or who are medically unfit for, radical cystectomy.

ADVANCED AND METASTATIC BLADDER CANCER

Transitional cell carcinoma can spread to the organs around the bladder (i.e., T4 or D1 disease), to the lymph nodes around the bladder (N+ or D1 disease), or it may metastasize to distant organs, most commonly liver, lung, or bone (M+ or D2 disease). At diagnosis, approximately 75 percent of patients will appear to have TCC confined to their bladder (i.e., Ta, Tis, T1, T2, or T3a), 20 percent will appear to have local spread of their disease outside the bladder (i.e., T3b or T4), and 5 percent of patients will present with findings of metastatic disease. However, approximately 50 percent of patients with muscle-invasive TCC treated with radical cystectomy will subsequently develop metastatic disease (usually within one year of their surgery). Survival rates in patients with metastatic bladder cancer are dismal with the average survival in untreated patients being less than twelve months, and nearly all of these patients dying of their cancer within two years.

Currently, the only treatment option that has shown any survival benefit in advanced bladder cancer is systemic chemotherapy with three- or four-drug combinations. The most effective multi-agent therapy to date appears to be M-VAC (i.e., methotrexate, vinblastine, adriamycin, and cis-platin). Patients are given various doses of these drugs intravenously. After receiving each drug once, the patients are given time to let the agents take effect and to allow their bodies and blood counts to recuperate from the effects of the chemotherapy. Then, another course, or cycle, of drugs is administered. Four cycles of therapy appear to be the minimum required to achieve "durable" responses.

Side effects of M-VAC can be substantial. The most common side effects include ulcerations in the mouth, nausea and vomiting, hair loss, low blood counts which can result in life-threatening infections, and kidney damage.

Complete responses to M-VAC have been reported in 40 percent of patients, and partial responses have also been reported for an overall response rate of approximately 60 to 70 percent. Unfortunately, the duration of these responses has been short (e.g., six to ten months). However, with these new chemotherapy regimens, five-year survival rates of 35 percent have been reported in patients with distant metastases. Long-term cures, however, are still infrequent.

Other chemotherapeutic regimens have been used in an attempt to achieve response rates similar to those with M-VAC but with decreased morbidity, one example being CMV (i.e., cis-platin, methotrexate, and vinblastine). Despite much study, at present, no curative treatment exists for advanced bladder cancer.

Avoiding bladder cancer requires action on two fronts: 1) patient, heal thyself –so, if you smoke, stop, and if you don't smoke, don't start; and 2) eternal vigilance –since these cancers tend to recur, close follow-up with a urologist is recommended. In those cases where the cancers progress to muscle-invasive disease, it can hopefully be caught early and at a time when radical cystectomy may save the patient's life.

References

1. Gillenwater JY, Grayhack JT, Howards SS, and Duckett JW (eds.): Adult and Pediatric Urology, 3rd ed. St. Louis: Mosby, 1996.
2. Korman HJ, Watson RB, and Soloway MS: "Bladder Cancer: Clinical Aspects and Management." *Monographs in Urology* 1996; 17(6):83-110.
3. Lamm DL and Lamm DA: "Superficial Bladder Cancer." *Urology Grand Rounds* 1997; 1(2):1-7.
4. Macfarlane MT: *Urology for the House Officer*, 2nd ed. Baltimore: Williams and Wilkins, 1995.

CHAPTER 23

KIDNEY CANCER

The kidneys are a pair of bean-shaped, reddish-brown organs, about 11 to 13 cm long, situated in the back part of the upper abdomen, lying alongside the spinal column, against the muscles of the back (see Figure 23-1). They function to filter and clean the blood of toxic substances. Each kidney receives its blood supply from the major artery in the body, known as the aorta, via the renal artery, and after filtering it returns the "purified" blood back to the main vein in the body, known as the inferior vena cava (IVC), via the renal vein. The toxic substances filtered by the kidneys are excreted into the urine, then pass, via the ureters, into the bladder, and are eventually eliminated from the body when the patient urinates.

Most people have one renal artery and one renal vein per kidney, but approximately 25 percent of people have more than one of these vessels supplying their kidneys. Accessory renal vessels are normal variants and usually are of no significance, except that the surgeon needs to consider the possibility of their presence when operating on the kidney. A suprarenal gland, also known as an adrenal gland, is located immediately above each kidney. These glands make hormones that are essential for survival. Around each kidney and adrenal gland is a layer of fat, called the perinephric fat, which is contained by a thin layer of fibrous tissue, called Gerota's fascia. Gerota's fascia separates the kidney, adrenal gland, and perinephric fat from the muscles of the back and the organs of the abdominal cavity.

It's possible to survive with one kidney and one adrenal gland. In fact, about one out of every 500 to 1000 persons are born with only one kidney. However, it is not possible to live without any kidneys and removal of both would require dialysis and/or a kidney transplant for the person to survive.

At times, cells in the kidney can become abnormal and develop into a kidney cancer.

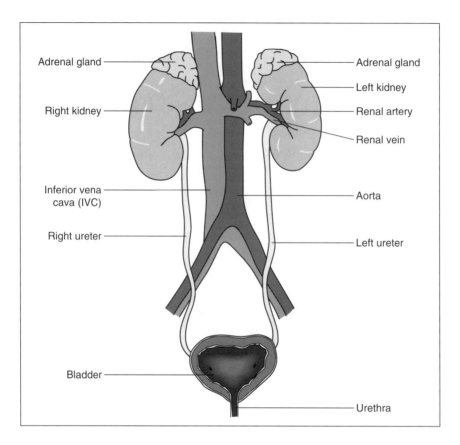

Figure 23-1: *Diagram of the urinary system; showing the adrenal gland (or suprarenal gland) and its relationship to the kidney.*

It should be noted that not all kidney masses are cancerous. In fact, the most common renal masses found are cysts. Renal cysts are fluid-filled sacs that develop in the kidney, and are present in up to 50 percent of patients over 50 years of age. They are benign and usually of no clinical significance except that they may achieve large sizes and cause the patient discomfort. The problem is that some renal cancers have cystic areas, although most renal cancers are composed of solid tissue. To add to the confusion, solid masses in the kidney may be benign or malignant. Unfortunately, the differentiation between these two often requires pathologic examination —the mass must be removed surgically and be examined by the pathologist to make a final diagnosis. Approximately 90 percent of all solid renal masses will be found to be cancerous. It should also be noted that there are many different cell types in the kidney which can give rise to different types of kidney cancer, but since approximately 90 percent of malignant renal tumors are renal cell carcinoma (RCC), this chapter will deal specifically with this type of kidney cancer.

Renal cell carcinoma, also known as hypernephroma or renal adeno-carcinoma, represents about 2 to 3 percent of all adult cancers, and is responsible for approximately 30,000 new cases and 12,000 deaths each year in the United States. RCC has been reported in children as young as six months of age, but the majority of patients diagnosed with this disease are 40 to 60 years old, with men twice as likely to get it. RCC usually occurs in only one kidney, and except in certain inherited diseases, bilateral RCC is very rare (i.e., less than 2 percent).

The cause of renal cell carcinoma remains unclear; however, certain factors have been associated with an increased risk of developing this type of cancer:

1. Cigarette smoking: Studies have suggested that cigarette smoking may increase a person's risk of developing RCC by two to three times over non-smokers.

2. Obesity and/or high fat diet.

3. Asbestos exposure.

4. Genetic abnormalities: RCC has been associated with a number of inherited disorders, and it is believed that certain genetic abnormalities (abnormalities in a person's DNA) may predispose a person to renal cell carcinoma.

DIAGNOSIS

Renal cell carcinoma may present itself in a variety of ways but, due to the location of the kidneys deep within the upper abdomen, RCC tends to grow silently and unnoticed, usually causing no symptoms, until it has progressed to an advanced stage. Years ago, before diagnostic studies, such as ultrasound or CT scan, the classic triad of flank pain, flank or abdominal mass, and hematuria was not only pathognomonic for RCC but also generally indicated advanced disease. Today, however, most renal cell carcinomas are diagnosed incidentally by ultrasound or CT scan in patients undergoing an evaluation for other problems, and only 10 percent of patients with RCC present with the "classic triad."

History

RCC is usually silent until the tumor achieves a large size or progresses far beyond the kidney. However, some symptoms that patients may complain of include:

1. Hematuria, either gross or microscopic, which is the most common presenting symptom or sign of RCC (found in up to 60 percent of patients).
2. A mass in the upper abdomen (20 to 45 percent).
3. Flank pain (35 to 40 percent).
4. Weight loss (28 to 36 percent).
5. Fever (7 to 17 percent).
6. Bone pain from spread of this cancer to the bones.

Physical Examination

The physical examination of patients with RCC is usually unremarkable. High blood pressure may be found in 20 to 40 percent of these patients. Occasionally, an upper-quadrant or flank mass may be palpated if the tumor achieves a large size.

Laboratory Studies

Various laboratory tests are performed in the evaluation of patients suspected of having a renal tumor:

Urinalysis (U/A)

Examination of the urine may reveal hematuria in up to 60 percent of patients with RCC. As stated in Chapter 18, hematuria requires further evaluation which may reveal a renal mass.

Complete Blood Count (CBC)

Approximately 20 to 40 percent of patients with RCC will be found to have anemia. On the other hand, 3 to 4 percent of patients with RCC have been reported to have an elevated red blood cell count, a condition known as erythrocytosis.

Serum Creatinine Level

In order to evaluate the patient's renal function before performing any x-ray studies, and before making any treatment recommendations, a blood test to check the patient's creatinine level is usually performed. Creatinine is a by-product of metabolism that is filtered and excreted almost exclusively by the kidneys. Therefore, as kidney function declines, creatinine accumulates in the blood, and the serum creatinine level rises. A normal serum creatinine level is less than 1.5 mg/dL, but levels less than 2 mg/dL are tolerable. Creatinine levels greater than 3 to 4 mg/dL may require dialysis.

Liver Function Tests (LFTs)

There are certain blood tests that help to evaluate the function of a person's liver (i.e., liver function tests, or LFTs). These blood tests may also be performed to evaluate patients for the possible spread of RCC to the liver; however, 10 to 15 percent of patients with RCC will have abnormal LFTs without evidence of metastatic liver disease, a condition known as Stauffer's syndrome. In the absence of metastatic disease to the liver, these laboratory values usually normalize after definitive treatment of the kidney cancer.

Serum Calcium Level

Approximately 3 to 6 percent of patients with renal cancer are found to have elevated blood levels of calcium believed to be due to hormone-like substances secreted by some of these cancers.

Special Studies

When the diagnosis of a kidney tumor is suspected, various confirmatory studies may be recommended.

Intravenous Pyelogram (IVP)

This is an x-ray study in which an iodine-based contrast material, injected intravenously, is filtered and excreted by the kidneys, allowing pictures to be taken of the kidneys, ureters, and bladder. IVP is still the most common initial diagnostic modality in the search for a renal mass, especially when patients present with hematuria. If a renal mass is seen on IVP, the next question that needs to be answered is whether the mass is cystic or solid. As noted earlier, the majority of renal masses seen on IVP are benign renal cysts, present in up to 50 percent of people over the age of 50. However, an IVP cannot make the distinction between cystic and solid lesions. Therefore, any renal mass found on IVP is usually evaluated further by ultrasound. For more details regarding IVP, please see Chapter 18.

Ultrasound of the Kidneys

In this study, sound waves are focused on the kidneys to take pictures of these structures. Ultrasound (U/S) is extremely accurate in differentiating cystic and solid elements. Masses that meet all the criteria for a benign cyst are called simple cysts and require no further follow-up or management as long as they are asymptomatic. Masses that are seen to be solid, complex (meaning mixtures of both cystic and solid elements), or indeterminate (meaning that they cannot be distinguished on ultrasound) require further evaluation with either CT scan or MRI.

Computed Axial Tomography Scan (CT scan)

This is an x-ray study during which the patient lies on a table which is passed through a circular machine that, with the help of a computer, makes cross-sectional images of the body. Since an iodine-based contrast solution is administered intravenously to help visualize certain structures, the risks of CT scan are similar to those for IVP (see Chapter 18). Urologists may recommend that a patient undergo a CT scan of the abdomen to further evaluate a renal mass found in the work-up of hematuria or other urologic symptoms. Urologists are also frequently asked to see patients with renal masses diagnosed incidentally by CT scan of the abdomen performed for other reasons, such as vague abdominal symptoms. In fact, as noted earlier, today most renal masses are found incidentally in the evaluation of other problems.

CT scan is very helpful in the diagnosis and staging of kidney cancer. It can provide information about the size and location of the mass as well as involvement of adjacent structures and lymph node or metastatic spread.

Magnetic Resonance Imaging Scan (MRI)

This study requires that the patient lie still for 30 to 40 minutes in a tube-shaped chamber that uses magnetic waves, instead of x-rays, to take pictures of the patient's internal organs. MRI is as accurate as, or slightly better than, CT scan in the diagnosis and staging of renal cell carcinoma. One advantage of MRI is that, unlike CT scan, it can be used in patients with poor renal function since no iodine-based contrast solution is required. One disadvantage of MRI is that people who are claustrophobic may not be able to tolerate the closed quarters for the time required to complete the study. Currently, MRI is most commonly used as an adjunct to, or in place of, the contrast CT scan.

Fine Needle Aspiration (FNA)

Rarely, an accurate diagnosis cannot be made from any of the above studies. In this case, the physician may recommend passing a needle into the kidney mass under local anesthesia in an attempt to obtain cells for microscopic examination using CT scan for guidance. FNA has a diagnostic accuracy of greater than 80 percent. If cancer is found in the biopsy specimen, further definitive treatment is indicated. If no cancer is found, follow-up with a repeat CT scan or MRI in three to six months is usually recommended. Even after an extensive evaluation, a definite diagnosis may not be possible, requiring surgical exploration and/or removal of the mass to make the diagnosis.

STAGING

Stage refers to the degree of invasion, or in other words, how far the tumor has spread into the surrounding tissues or to other parts of the body, if at all. Physicians use various special studies, especially CT scan or MRI, to estimate the stage of a kidney tumor, known as the clinical stage (as opposed to the pathologic stage which is determined after the specimen is removed surgically and examined by the pathologist). Accurate clinical staging, combined with other data available at the time of diagnosis (e.g., the patient's overall health), helps the urologist assess the patient's prognosis and make rational treatment recommendations.

CT scan is the most commonly employed modality in the diagnosis and staging of renal tumors. MRI may be necessary in patients who cannot receive intravenous contrast agents or in whom the CT scan findings are equivocal. Some additional staging studies that may be suggested include:

- Chest x-ray (CXR): This study may be used to search for the spread of RCC to the lungs.

- Bone scan: This is a study in which a radioactive solution is injected intravenously. The radioactive material, or tracer, accumulates in areas of bone involved with cancer, and will show up on a machine that detects radioactivity. Other conditions that can cause bone to accumulate radioactive tracer, and thus which may confuse this finding on bone scan, include: arthritis, old fractures, and infections in the bone. Bone scans are not routinely performed in the work-up of a possible renal cancer, unless the patient complains of bone pain or certain laboratory studies are abnormal.

There are two staging systems in common use for RCC: the Robson system (see Figure 23-2), and the international TNM system which stands for T - tumor, N - nodes (or lymph node involvement), and M - metastases (or distant spread of the cancer).

In the Robson system:

- **Stage I** cancers are confined to the kidney.

- **Stage II** tumors have broken through the renal capsule (i.e., the outer lining of the kidney) to get outside the kidney into the perinephric fat or adrenal gland, but are contained within Gerota's fascia.

- **Stage IIIa** cancers extend into the renal vein or IVC (inferior vena cava).

- **Stage IIIb** tumors involve the local lymph nodes.

- **Stage IIIc** disease involves *both* the renal vein or IVC *and* local lymph nodes.

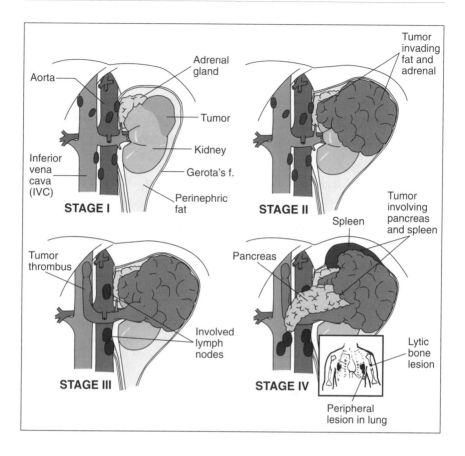

Figure 23-2: *Robson Staging System for RCC (From Gillenwater JY, et al., Adult and Pediatric Urology, 3rd ed. St. Louis: Mosby, 1996; as adapted from Robson CJ, Churchill BM, Anderson W: "The Results of Radical Nephrectomy for Renal Cell Carcinoma." J Urol 1969, 101:297.*

- **Stage IV** tumors invade adjacent organs (other than the adrenal glands) or have metastasized to distant sites (most commonly to lung, liver, bone, or brain).

In the TNM system:

- **T1** tumors are confined to the kidney but are not larger than 2.5 cm in diameter.
- **T2** cancers are confined to the kidney but are larger than 2.5 cm in diameter.

- **T3a** tumors extend beyond the renal capsule but are confined within Gerota's fascia.

- **T3b** cancers extend into the renal vein.

- **T3c** tumors involve the renal vein and IVC.

- **T4** tumors invade adjacent tissues or organs beyond Gerota's fascia.

- **N0** signifies that no lymph nodes around the kidney are involved with cancer.

- **N1** denotes that cancer has spread to one lymph node which is not larger than 2 cm.

- **N2** denotes cancer spread to 1 or more lymph nodes, all totaling more than 2 cm and less than 5 cm in size.

- **N3** signifies that the cancer spread in the local lymph nodes has achieved a size of 5 cm or larger.

- **M0** signifies that the cancer does not appear to have spread to distant organs.

- **M1** denotes that the cancer has spread far beyond the kidney (e.g., to the lungs, liver, bones, or brain).

A comparison of the two staging systems is seen in Table 23-1.

A definitive diagnosis of RCC cannot be made without pathologic examination of a tissue specimen, but with the development of CT scan and other modalities, such as MRI, and given the fact that 90 percent of solid renal masses are cancerous, usually renal cell carcinomas, urologists can usually make a tentative diagnosis of RCC before any invasive studies. Once it is determined that the patient has, or most probably has, a renal cancer, the urologist usually discusses the various treatment options available and makes recommendations for the treatment of the patient's cancer. These recommendations are usually based on many pieces of information, some of which include: the age and general health of the patient, the likelihood that the cancer is confined to the kidney (i.e., the clinical stage of disease), and the information regarding the success rates of the various treatment options available at the time of diagnosis. The patient may be given some time to think about his options before making a final decision as to how he wants his kidney cancer to be treated.

Table 23-1:
Summary of the TNM and Robson Staging Systems

TNM	Robson	What the Results Mean:
T0	-	No cancer present.
T1	I	Tumor is confined to the kidney (< 2.5 cm.).
T2	I	Tumor is confined to the kidney (> 2.5 cm.).
T3a	II	Tumor extends beyond the renal capsule but is confined within Gerota's fascia.
T3b	IIIa	Tumor extends into the renal vein.
T3c	IIIa	Tumor involves the renal vein and IVC.
T4	IV	Tumor invades adjacent tissue or organs beyond Gerota's fascia.
N0	-	No lymph nodes involved by cancer.
N1	IIIb	Cancer has spread to one lymph node 2 cm. or smaller.
N2	IIIb	Cancer has spread to 1 or more lymph nodes, totaling between 2-5 cm. in size.
N3	IIIb	Cancer in the lymph nodes has achieved a size of more than 5 cm.
M0	-	No distant spread of disease.
M1	IV	Cancer has spread far beyond the kidney (e.g., to the lungs, liver, bones or brain).

TREATMENT OPTIONS

Surgery

Surgical removal is presently the only known effective treatment modality for localized renal cell carcinoma. It may involve excision of the entire kidney or removal of only that part of the kidney containing the tumor. Before surgery, there are a few steps that may be taken in an attempt to optimize conditions for the procedure:

1. It is recommended that the patient stop using aspirin, ibuprofen, or other products that can thin their blood, at least one week before surgery to try to prevent excessive bleeding during or after the procedure.

2. Since some patients lose enough blood to require a transfusion during or after the operation, in the weeks before their surgery, patients may be asked to donate their own blood for the specific purpose of having

it available in case they need a transfusion during or after the surgery. This technique is called autologous blood donation. In addition, there are machines which can collect the blood lost during surgery. After processing, this blood can be transfused back into the patient in an attempt to avoid the need for transfusion of blood from the blood bank.

3. The patient is advised not to eat or drink anything after midnight the night before surgery.

Radical Nephrectomy

Radical nephrectomy involves removal of the kidney and ipsilateral adrenal gland together with the perinephric fat, Gerota's fascia, and local lymph nodes. The patient is usually admitted to the hospital on the morning of the procedure which is typically performed under general anesthesia. The approach to the kidney cancer depends on the size of the tumor, the patient's body habitus (i.e., the patient's build or size), and surgeon preference; however, the incision will usually be made either in the patient's flank with him lying on his side (sometimes requiring removal of a rib), or anteriorly in the upper abdomen just below the patient's rib cage on the affected side. Once dissection is performed and the kidney is exposed, the blood vessels to the kidney and adrenal gland are tied off, and the kidney and adrenal gland are dissected free from surrounding structures. The ureter is also tied off and transected. Then, the kidney, adrenal gland, perinephric fat, and Gerota's fascia are removed and sent to the pathologist for examination and pathologic staging.

Tumor may be found extending into the renal vein (15 to 20 percent of cases) or IVC (5 to 10 percent), and this will require removal as well, sometimes with the aid of heart bypass machines. Local lymph nodes are also usually removed for staging purposes. Whether the removal of local lymph nodes involved with cancer helps prolong survival is controversial.

The operation usually takes about two hours. After the procedure, the patient is given pain medication to keep him as comfortable as possible, and his diet is advanced as tolerated. The usual hospital stay is between three and five days, but every patient reacts differently to surgery. The patient generally returns to the office seven days after his surgery to have the staples removed from his skin incision. Patients are advised not to drive for one to two weeks and to avoid strenuous activity for four to six weeks. Walking, however, is encouraged.

Follow-up after surgery tends to depend on the pathologic stage of disease. If it appears that the cancer has been completely excised, the patient is followed regularly by his urologist, with laboratory studies and a chest x-ray every three to six months for a few years and then yearly for a few more years. He also may undergo a yearly CT scan of the abdomen to search for recurrent disease. If the patient survives five years after surgery without evidence of recurrent tumor, he is usually considered cured. If the pathology report suggests that residual cancer may exist, additional treatment options are discussed with the patient.

The overall complication rate of radical nephrectomy is approximately 2 percent. Some of the reported complications include:

1. Infection.

2. Bleeding which may require transfusion: Again, the steps described prior have decreased the need for transfusion of blood from the blood bank; however, there is still a rare possibility that the patient may lose enough blood to require a transfusion of banked blood. Blood is now screened for the presence of hepatitis and AIDS, so although there are still risks associated with banked blood, they are low.

3. Pain: Various medications are used in the post-operative period to try to keep the patient as comfortable as possible. Patients are also given a prescription for oral pain medication to take at home for two to three weeks after their surgery.

4. Hernia: The sutures used to close the muscles and tissues deep inside the patient can break with strenuous activity resulting in a hernia. Therefore, patients are advised to avoid strenuous activity for four to six weeks after surgery. Of note, after being transected (or cut with a knife), the muscles of the body wall can become weak causing a bulge to develop in the area of the incision. This phenomenon, which can be perceived by the patient to be a hernia, is known as a flank bulge.

5. Renal failure: People can survive with only one kidney, as long as the remaining kidney functions normally. After losing one kidney, most patients experience a decline in renal function, as evidenced by a slight

increase in their serum creatinine level. Rarely, this decline in renal function may be so severe as to require temporary or permanent dialysis to support the function of the remaining kidney. In an attempt to avoid this complication, if the patient's kidney function is tenuous before surgery, a procedure to spare as much functioning renal tissue as possible is usually recommended (i.e., partial nephrectomy).

6. Damage to adjacent structures: Nearby organs that may be injured during this operation include the liver, intestines, spleen, blood vessels, various nerves, and the lung cavity (a condition known as pneumothorax).

7. Pneumonia: Patients are encouraged to perform deep breathing exercises after their operation to decrease their risk of developing this problem.

8. Prolonged ileus: This condition involves a delay in the return of intestinal function and can be manifested as abdominal bloating, nausea, or vomiting.

9. Deep vein thrombosis (DVT) and/or pulmonary embolus (PE): During this procedure, the patient lies on the operating table for two to three hours while the urologist operates around major blood vessels in the body. As a result, clots can form in the veins that drain the legs, a condition known as DVT. Sometimes, these clots can break free and travel through the bloodstream to lodge in the lungs, a condition known as a PE, which can be fatal.

10. Residual or recurrent tumor: After the operation, the pathology report may suggest residual cancer, but patients are also followed regularly to search for evidence of recurrent disease.

11. Removal of the kidney for a benign tumor: Benign tumors comprise approximately 5 to 10 percent of solid renal masses. Unfortunately, since it is often impossible to differentiate benign solid masses from renal cancers, and since solid renal masses are considered to be malignant until proven otherwise, it usually requires radical nephrectomy to make the final diagnosis.

12. Heart attack and/or death (2 percent).

Radical nephrectomy is indicated in generally healthy patients with solid renal masses, suspected of being RCC, that appear confined to the kidney and/or renal vein or IVC, and who have a normal-functioning contralateral kidney.

Partial Nephrectomy

In general, this procedure involves removal of only that part of the kidney containing the cancer in an attempt to preserve as much functioning kidney tissue as possible while ridding the patient of his cancer. The preparation of the patient and the surgical approach to the kidney is usually similar to that for patients undergoing radical nephrectomy.

Once the kidney is exposed, the tumor mass is localized. A variety of surgical techniques have been described to perform partial nephrectomy, but generally, a wedge of tissue, including the tumor mass and a margin of normal-appearing renal tissue, is excised and sent to the pathologist for examination and confirmation that the margins of resection are free of tumor.

The operation usually takes about two to three hours. The patient may have a drainage tube placed around the kidney and brought out to the skin through a separate smaller incision near the larger cut, to prevent the accumulation of blood and/or urine inside the patient. This drain is removed when its output is minimal, usually around the second or third post-operative day. After the procedure, the patient is managed with pain medication, and his diet is advanced as tolerated. The usual hospital stay is four to five days. The patient usually returns to the office to have his skin staples removed about seven days after the surgery.

Post-operative advice and follow-up are similar to those for patients undergoing radical nephrectomy.

The complications seen after partial nephrectomy are similar to those seen after radical nephrectomy. In addition, complications specific to partial nephrectomy include:

1. Urinary fistula: This is a connection between the urinary tract and the skin and is manifested as prolonged flank drainage. The majority of these fistulas will heal spontaneously; however, invasive procedures may be required if conservative treatment fails.

2. Ureteral obstruction: Scarring from surgery can result in narrowing or occlusion of the ureter which may require further intervention.

3. Renal failure: Varying degrees of renal insufficiency occur after partial nephrectomy, depending on the patient's degree of renal function pre-operatively and the amount of functioning renal tissue removed. If severe, this renal dysfunction may require temporary dialysis (7 percent), or may progress to permanent renal failure requiring permanent dialysis (3 percent).

4. Need for radical nephrectomy: Occasionally, due to bleeding or the inability to achieve tumor-free margins, the entire kidney may need to be removed during the surgery, and this may result in the need for permanent dialysis as well.

5. Residual or recurrent tumor: The risk of this occurring in small RCC's (i.e., less than 3 cm in diameter) is approximately 2 percent, but in larger tumors, this risk may be as high as 10 percent.

Although radical nephrectomy remains the treatment of choice for the patient with localized renal cell carcinoma and a normal opposite kidney, partial nephrectomy is the treatment of choice when localized RCC is present in both kidneys, in a patient with only one kidney, or in patients with poor renal function (i.e., creatinine level is higher than 2) or in patients with a disease that may threaten the function of the remaining kidney in the future, such as diabetes or kidney stones.

Radiation Therapy

Radiation has been used pre-operatively and post-operatively as an adjunct to surgical treatment. In this form of therapy, x-rays are focused on the area around the kidney to try to destroy residual cancer cells. Survival has not been shown to be enhanced in most studies. Radiation therapy can be beneficial in relieving discomfort when used to treat patients with pain from RCC that has metastasized to the bones. In these cases, the x-rays are focused on the sites of metastasis.

Chemotherapy

Various chemotherapeutic drugs have been tried in patients with metastatic RCC; however, to date, the results of chemotherapy for advanced RCC have been disappointing with only 5 to 10 percent of patients responding to treatment for only short periods of time.

Hormonal Therapy

Estrogen, progesterone, and other hormones have been used in metastatic renal cancer in an attempt to inhibit tumor growth and progression. However, hormone therapy appears to be ineffective against RCC, with partial response rates of only 1 to 2 percent.

Immunotherapy

This form of treatment involves the administration of various agents in an attempt to stimulate the patient's own immune system to fight his kidney cancer. It has usually been used in patients with advanced or metastatic RCC, with or without radical nephrectomy. The exact mechanism of action and the optimum treatment regimens of the various agents are unclear. Some of the immunotherapeutic agents used to treat RCC have included interferon and interleukin-2.

Side effects reported with some of these agents include: fever, fatigue, nausea, vomiting, diarrhea, high blood pressure, liver damage, and heart attack.

Reported response rates have been between 10 and 30 percent with an average duration of responses of four to twelve months.

Although immunotherapy appears to be more effective than other systemic modalities for metastatic RCC, further studies are needed to develop more effective and less toxic forms of therapy for advanced stages of this disease.

TREATMENT BY STAGE

Stages I and II

Radical nephrectomy is the standard and the only effective treatment option for localized RCC. Reported five-year survival rates for Robson stage I tumors have been 60 to 90 percent, and those for stage II tumors are 50 to 80 percent. Unfortunately, approximately 50 percent of patients treated with surgery will eventually develop signs of metastatic disease. Patients with bilateral RCC, cancer in a solitary kidney, or poor renal function are usually advised to undergo a partial nephrectomy, if feasible.

Stage III

Patients with only renal vein or inferior vena cava (IVC) extension appear to benefit from radical nephrectomy. Local lymph node involvement is a poor prognostic sign, but since radical nephrectomy is the only effective therapy for RCC, radical surgery, with or without subsequent immuno-therapy, may be an option if lymph node involvement is found at the time of surgery. Five-year survival rates for stage III tumors without lymph node involvement have been reported to be 50 to 60 percent, whereas those for patients with stage III RCC with lymph node involvement have been reported to be approximately 15 to 25 percent.

Stage IV

Distant metastatic disease is present in 20 percent of patients at the time of diagnosis. In addition, 50 percent of patients treated with radical surgery for apparent clinically-localized disease will develop signs of metastatic cancer at a later date. These patients have an average survival of four months, and only 10 percent survive one year. Although a few studies have reported regression of metastatic deposits after radical nephrectomy (a situation which may occur in less than 1 percent of cases), nephrectomy in this stage is usually reserved for the palliative treatment of severe bleeding that cannot be stopped by other means, pain, or other significant symptoms attributable to the renal cancer itself.

As seen in the previous section, radiation therapy, chemotherapy, and hormone therapy offer no significant survival benefit in the management of metastatic renal cell carcinoma; however, immunotherapy may be of benefit in treating this stage of disease. Protocols involving experimental therapy are usually carried out at university medical centers; therefore, patients with advanced RCC seeking additional treatment options may want to consider further evaluation at university medical centers or cancer centers in their area.

PROGNOSIS

The stage of the cancer at the time of surgical exploration is the most important prognostic indicator for the patient with renal cell carcinoma. Survival decreases in patients with increasing stage, with only 5 to 10 percent of patients with distant metastatic disease at the time of diagnosis surviving five years. Extension of tumor into the renal vein or IVC does not appear to have a significant impact on survival, as long as the tumor is confined within Gerota's fascia, no evidence of lymph node involvement or distant spread is found, and all tumor can be removed from the IVC. Table 23-2 summarizes the prognosis of patients with RCC based on the stage of their disease.

Table 23-2: Prognosis of Patients Treated for RCC Based on the Stage of the Disease	
Robson Stage	**5-Year Survival (%)**
I	60-90
II	50-80
III (renal vein or IVC)	50-60
III (lymph node +)	15-25
IV	5-10

Modified from: Gillenwater et al.,*Adult and Pediatric Urology, 3rd ed.* St. Louis: Mosby, 1996.

At the present time, surgery is the only effective treatment option for localized RCC, and although experiments with immunotherapy are promising, the prognosis for patients with advanced renal cell carcinoma remains poor.

References

1. Davis BE and Weigel JW: "Management of Advanced Renal Cell Carcinoma." *AUA Update Series* 1990; vol. 9, lesson 3.
2. Gardner E, Gray DJ, and O'Rahilly R: *Anatomy*, 4th ed. Philadelphia: Saunders, 1975.
3. Gillenwater JY, Grayhack JT, Howards SS, and Duckett JW (eds.): *Adult and Pediatric Urology*, 3rd ed. St. Louis: Mosby, 1996.
4. Hollinshead WH, and Rosse C: *Textbook of Anatomy*, 4th ed., Philadelphia: Harper and Row Publishers, 1985.
5. Macfarlane MT: *Urology for the House Officer*, 2nd ed. Baltimore: Williams and Wilkins, 1995.
6. Sokoloff MH, Figlin RA, and Belldegrun AS: "Management of Metastatic Renal Cell Carcinoma." *AUA Update Series* 1996; vol. 15, lesson 30.

CHAPTER 24

TESTICULAR CANCER

Chapter 17 discussed the anatomy of the scrotum and some of the more common causes of scrotal masses. This chapter will focus on one of those causes —namely, testicular cancer. Many different cell types in the testicle can become cancerous, but 95 to 97 percent of all testicular malignancies arise from cells involved in reproduction known as the germ cells. This chapter will exclusively address this particular type of testicular cancer, also called *germ cell tumors.*

Testicular cancer is seen in approximately 2 out of every 100,000 males. Although they are rare, testicular cancers are the most common solid tumors seen in young adult men, with approximately 5000 new cases and 1000 deaths reported each year in the United States. Testicular tumors have been reported in males from infancy to age 89, but most frequently occur in men between the ages of 15 and 40. They are more common in whites than in nonwhites, and tend to occur slightly more often in the right testicle than in the left. Testicular cancers rarely occur bilaterally (2 to 3 percent of all cases), and when they do, it is not necessarily at the same time.

As with other malignancies, the cause of testicular cancer remains unknown. One factor believed to increase the risk of developing a testicular cancer is an undescended testicle. Approximately 10 percent of patients who develop a testicular cancer report having had an undescended testicle, and in 50 percent of these patients, the undescended testicle was located in the abdominal cavity. It should be noted that today it is recommended that most undescended testicles be surgically placed into the scrotum, using a variety of techniques, when the child is one to two years of age. This surgery may help the future reproductive function of the testicle, but it does not appear to decrease the risk of developing a testicular cancer in these patients. In addition, for some unknown reason, this risk of testicular cancer appears to include the other testicle, since in approximately 20 percent of patients with testicular cancer and a history of an undescended testicle, the cancer developed in the contralateral normally descended testicle.

Problems with the immune system may also increase a person's risk of developing testicular cancer. In fact, testicular tumors are 20 to 50 times more common in immunosuppressed patients and those who have had organ transplants than in the general population. It was once thought that trauma to the testicle might increase the risk of developing a testicular malignancy. Most authors now believe that trauma does not predispose the testicle to cancer, but rather that the trauma is the event that prompts the evaluation of the testicle, leading to the discovery of the cancer.

DIAGNOSIS

History

Patients with a testicular cancer most commonly complain of a scrotal swelling, so although most scrotal masses are benign, any patient who discovers himself to have a scrotal mass should seek further medical evaluation. Patients have also reported a fullness or "heavy-feeling" in the scrotum. On rare occasions, patients may present with signs of advanced disease, such as weight loss or an abdominal mass. Hormones released by certain testicular cancers may result in swelling of the patient's breast tissue, a condition known as gynecomastia.

Since approximately 10 percent of patients with testicular cancer will have an initial presentation similar to epididymitis (see Chapter 15), in order to avoid a significant delay in diagnosis, it is recommended that patients diagnosed with epididymitis follow-up with their doctor after treatment to make sure that the epididymitis has resolved and that no residual scrotal masses are present.

Physical Examination

An examination of the genitalia by an experienced physician is a crucial part of the evaluation of a scrotal mass; however, campaigns for testicular self-examination have had an impact on earlier detection of testicular cancer. Therefore, frequent self-examination (e.g., every one to two months) has been recommended for men at risk (i.e., those between 15 and

45 years of age). The examination can be performed in the shower, just before dressing, or immediately after disrobing, and usually takes only a few minutes. Two hands are used to examine one testicle at a time. One hand steadies the testicle, and the other hand grasps it, using the fingertips and the tip of the thumb to try to feel any masses. The normal testicle is smooth and feels like a hard-boiled egg without its shell. Any lumps, bumps, or hard areas in the testicle could be a testicular cancer; therefore, if the self-examination reveals a possible mass or any change from a previous examination, or if a person has any questions regarding his self-examination, he should see a physician as soon as possible for further evaluation.

If the diagnosis of a testicular mass is confirmed by a physician, the patient will usually be referred to a urologist for further management. Some particular areas that might be examined by the urologist as part of the evaluation of a testicular mass include:

- Neck: for evidence of spread to the lymph nodes in the neck area.
- Chest: to search for evidence of gynecomastia.
- Abdomen: for evidence of a mass which would suggest the presence of advanced disease.
- Genitalia: to confirm the presence of a scrotal mass and attempt to differentiate intratesticular from extratesticular lesions.

Laboratory Studies

Urinalysis

A urinalysis (U/A) may be performed in patient's suspected of having an infection as the cause of their scrotal mass (e.g., epididymitis).

Tumor Markers

A tumor marker is a protein produced by a cancer which can be measured by a blood test in an attempt to detect that cancer. Two such tumor markers used in the evaluation of patients suspected of having a testicular cancer are beta-human chorionic gonadotropin (B-HCG) and alpha-feto-protein (AFP). Normally, these proteins are not present in large amounts in the bloodstream; however, either of these may be elevated in patients with testicular cancer. In fact, 70 percent of all testis tumors will produce one or more serum tumor markers. Although testicular cancers can be present despite normal levels of these tumor markers, abnormal elevations are highly suggestive for the presence of testicular cancer. Therefore, tests for serum tumor markers are usually obtained prior to surgical exploration in patients with a testicular mass. Physicians also monitor the levels of these tumor markers after treatment to help evaluate the patient's response to therapy and to detect the presence of residual or recurrent disease.

Liver Function Tests

Liver function tests (LFTs) are a group of blood tests used to screen for abnormalities in the liver. Patients whose cancer has spread to the liver may have abnormalities in these blood tests, so LFTs may be used to screen for the spread of testicular cancer to the liver.

Special Studies

Ultrasound

Ultrasound of the scrotum involves a machine that bounces sound waves off the testicles to make pictures of them and other structures in the scrotum. It is harmless and painless and usually takes only a few minutes to perform. Its ability to demonstrate whether a mass is located within the testicle is important, since most intratesticular masses are malignant, while most extratesticular masses are benign.

Occasionally, despite this extensive evaluation, it is not possible to satisfactorily determine whether or not a scrotal mass is a testicular mass. In these cases, the urologist may recommend surgical exploration and possible removal of the testicle if a cancer is found.

TREATMENT OF TESTICULAR TUMORS

If a solid mass is found to be located within, or arising from, the testicle itself, then surgical removal of the testicle via an incision in the inguinal, or groin, area is indicated.

The patient is admitted on the day of surgery, and the procedure is usually performed under general or spinal anesthesia. An incision is made in the inguinal area on the side of the testicular mass, and the testicle and spermatic cord (i.e., the group of blood vessels and nerves that supply the testicle) are dissected free from surrounding structures. If the mass definitely arises from the testicle itself, the spermatic cord is tied off and transected near its entrance into the abdominal cavity, and the testicle and spermatic cord are removed and sent to the pathologist for study. This operation is known as a radical orchiectomy.

As stated earlier, occasionally the diagnosis of a testicular mass cannot be made preoperatively with certainty. If this is the case, surgical exploration is performed via an inguinal incision, and the urologist examines the testicle under anesthesia. If it is still not possible to rule out a cancer, an intra-operative biopsy of the lesion can be performed and sent to the pathologist for immediate examination. If the lesion is found to be benign, the testicle may be replaced into the scrotum. If, however, the lesion is found to be cancerous, a radical orchiectomy is performed. In any equivocal case, a radical orchiectomy is usually performed, and the final diagnosis is made by the pathologist.

Radical orchiectomy usually lasts 30 to 60 minutes. Patients are sent home on the day of surgery or the following morning with oral pain medication. They are advised not to take any aspirin, ibuprofen, or other blood-thinners for a few weeks after the surgery to try to decrease the risk of post-operative bleeding. Patients are also advised to abstain from any strenuous activity for four to six weeks after the operation in an attempt to avoid developing a hernia at the incision site.

Radical orchiectomy is usually well tolerated. Complications are rare but may include:

1. Infection.
2. Bleeding: The most common complication reported after a radical orchiectomy is the collection of blood in the scrotum, known as a scrotal hematoma, which usually resolves spontaneously with conservative management.
3. Pain: Oral pain medication is usually adequate to keep patients comfortable after this procedure.
4. Hernia.

5. Possibility of removing a testicle for benign disease: Sometimes, the nature of a lesion in, on, or around the testicle cannot be determined by visual examination, and even a biopsy may be equivocal. In these cases, it may be prudent to perform a radical orchiectomy and have the pathologist make the final diagnosis.

6. Heart attack and/or death: These are risks associated with anesthesia, but they are rare in young, healthy patients.

After the operation, the specimen is sent to the pathologist for examination. In the rare cases when the tumor is found to be benign, the good news is relayed to the patient, and no further treatment or long-term follow-up is required. If the patient is found to have testicular cancer, the cell-type of the tumor and the stage (or degree of spread) of the patient's disease must be determined before additional treatment recommendations can be made.

CELL TYPE

Testicular cancers are generally divided into two groups based on the type of cells that make up the tumor: seminoma or nonseminoma. The distinction between seminomas and nonseminomas is made by a pathologist based on the microscopic appearances of these tumors. This classification developed due to the differences in the way these two groups respond to various treatments. Seminomas tend to be very responsive to radiation, while nonseminomatous tumors (NST) are very responsive to surgery and/or chemotherapy. It should be noted that tumors with mixtures of both seminoma and nonseminoma are usually managed as a NST.

STAGE

Stage refers to the degree of invasion, or in other words, how far the cancer has spread into the surrounding tissues or to other parts of the body, if at all. The stage of the patient's cancer is used to help the urologist assess the patient's prognosis and make rational treatment recommendations.

There are two staging systems currently in use: the more common, original ABC system of Boden and Gibb, modified by Skinner, and the international TNM classification, which stands for T - tumor, N - nodes (i.e., lymph node involvement), M - metastasis (i.e., distant spread of cancer).

Before discussing the staging systems further, it should be noted that the testicles do not originate in the scrotum. As seen in Figure 24-1, the testicles originate high in the back part of the abdomen, near the kidneys, and during the development of the fetus, they migrate downward, descending into the scrotum shortly before or after birth. Since the blood supply of each testicle originates at the level of the kidneys, any spread of testicular cancer to "local" lymph nodes occurs to those lymph nodes located at the origin of the blood supply of the testicle, which is situated at the level of the kidneys.

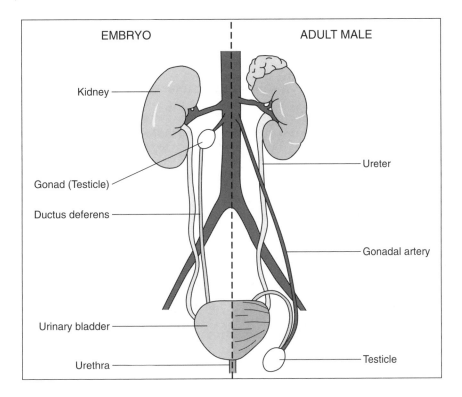

Figure 24-1: *Schematic representation of the development of the blood supply of the testicle and kidney. The testicle develops near the kidney (left half of the figure) . Later, the testicle descends, carrying its blood vessels with it. The right half of the figure demonstrates the anatomical relationships in the adult male.*

In the ABC system:

- **Stage A** signifies that the cancer is confined to the testicle.
- **Stage B** denotes that the cancer has spread to the local lymph nodes (also called the retroperitoneal lymph nodes).
    - B1 cancers involve less than 6 lymph nodes, and no lymph node is over 2 cm.
    - B2 cancers involve more than 6 lymph nodes, and the lymph nodes are 2 to 6 cm in size.
    - B3 cancers have massive retroperitoneal disease (i.e., the tumor mass involving the lymph nodes is greater than 6 cm in size).
- **Stage C** denotes distant spread of disease (e.g., to lungs, liver, brain, or bone).

In the TNM system:

- **T0** means that no tumor is found in the testicle.
- **T1** tumor is confined to the testicle.
- **T2** cancer has penetrated the outer lining of the testicle, called the *tunica albuginea*.
- **T3** cancers invade the tubules leading out of the testicle (i.e., the rete testis), or the epididymis.
- **T4a** cancers invade the structures of the spermatic cord.
- **T4b** tumors have invaded the scrotal wall.
- **N0** means that no lymph nodes are involved with cancer.
- **N1** signifies retroperitoneal lymph node spread involving only the nodes on the side of the testicular tumor.
- **N2** cancers involve the retroperitoneal lymph nodes on both sides of the patient.
- **N3** disease is so significant that the mass can be felt through the abdominal wall.
- **M0** signifies no evidence of distant spread.
- **M1** indicates that the cancer has spread to distant sites (e.g., lungs, liver, brain, or bone).

When comparing the two systems, any T stage would be fairly equivalent to stage A, although in the higher T stages, the tumor can be outside the testicle and still have no evidence of lymph node spread. N+ disease is equivalent to stage B, with further substaging based on the amount of disease in the retroperitoneal lymph nodes, and M+ disease is equivalent to stage C in the Boden-Gibb-Skinner system.

Various studies are used to clinically stage a person's testicular cancer, and are described below.

Repeat Tumor Markers

Persistent elevation of any tumor marker a few weeks after a radical orchiectomy is a sign of residual cancer which demands further treatment. It should be noted, however, that normal levels of tumor markers, although a good sign after surgery, do not assure that tumor is absent.

Chest X-ray

This test is used to search for evidence of the spread of testicular cancer to the patient's lungs. Small lesions may not be detectable.

Computed Axial Tomography Scan (CT Scan)

Computed axial tomography scan or CT scan is an x-ray study during which the patient lies on a table which is passed through a circular machine that, with the help of a computer, makes cross-sectional images of the body. It is used to search for enlarged retroperitoneal lymph nodes involved with testicular cancer. Since an iodine-based contrast solution is administered intravenously to help visualize certain structures, the risks of CT scan are similar to those of IVP (see Chapter 18). CT scan requires enlargement of the lymph nodes to detect involvement with cancer; therefore, it is unable to detect microscopic spread of disease to lymph nodes that fails to increase their size.

Magnetic Resonance Imaging Scan (MRI)

This study involves the use of magnetic waves, instead of x-rays, to take pictures of the patient's internal organs. Patients are required to lie still in a tube-shaped chamber for 30 to 40 minutes during the study, which may create a problem for claustrophobic patients. MRI can be used in place of CT scan to search for enlarged lymph nodes in the staging work-up of testicular cancer.

The overall accuracy of clinical staging is approximately 70 to 80 percent, which means that 20 to 30 percent of patients with lymph node spread or metastatic disease will have no evidence of such advanced disease, despite using the above studies.

Once the cell-type (seminoma vs. nonseminoma) and clinical stage of the patient's cancer have been determined, the urologist discusses the various treatment options available, and usually makes recommendations for the further management of the patient's disease.

TREATMENT OPTIONS AFTER ORCHIECTOMY

Testicular cancers tend to be fast-growing. As a result, disease is frequently found beyond the testicle at the time of diagnosis. Various treatment options exist to manage patients after radical orchiectomy.

Retroperitoneal Lymph Node Dissection (RPLND)

This operation helps to accurately stage patients by sampling the lymph nodes around the kidneys (to which testicular cancer may spread), but it is also used for the treatment of testicular cancer by allowing the surgeon to remove lymph nodes involved with cancer.

The patient is admitted to the hospital on the morning of the operation. With the patient under general anesthesia, an incision is made in the midline of the abdomen from just below the breast bone to just above the penis. The surgeon removes the lymph nodes around the kidney as well as the lymphatic tissue around the blood vessels that supplied the testicle on the side of the cancer. The extent of dissection depends on the amount of cancer in the lymph nodes, if any.

In the past, the standard RPLND resulted in infertility in a significant number of patients. Over the years, modifications in surgical technique have led to the development of the nerve-sparing RPLND, in which the nerves responsible for proper ejaculation can be spared, thus preserving ejaculatory function in 85 to 97 percent of patients. Since most patients who develop testicular cancer are in their reproductive years and might want to have children, these technical advances are significant.

RPLND usually lasts two to three hours. Post-operatively, patients are allowed liquids when alert, and their diets are advanced as tolerated. Patients are kept comfortable with pain medication. The typical hospital stay is four to seven days, and patients are usually given a prescription for pain medication to take at home. They are advised to avoid any strenuous activity for four to six weeks after the operation, and can usually return to work in a few weeks, depending on the type of work and the necessity for physical labor.

Some centers now perform RPLND using a laparoscopic approach. This procedure is performed under general anesthesia. A telescopic instrument is placed into the abdominal cavity through a small hole made near the belly-button. Then, using instruments placed into the abdominal cavity through several other small holes, the lymph nodes are removed in a manner similar to the open procedure. The laparoscopic method takes a little longer than open RPLND and requires a urologic surgeon trained in laparoscopic techniques, but the post-operative recovery period is much shorter.

Regardless of the approach, post-operative follow-up includes regular visits to the urologist, blood tests (e.g., serum AFP and B-HCG), and chest x-rays. Follow-up schedules vary, but visits are usually every one to three months for the first two years, then every six months for the next two years, then once-a-year for a few more years before the patient is considered cured. Patients found to have more tumor than expected from the pre-operative staging evaluation may require additional treatment which might also alter their follow-up schedule.

Some of the complications associated with RPLND include:

1. Infection (up to 15 percent): The risk of infection is greatest in patients who have received chemotherapy before surgery.

2. Bleeding: The need for transfusion during or after this operation is rare, especially since patients tend to be young and relatively healthy.

3. Pain: This is major surgery; however, post-operatively, patients are kept comfortable using a variety of intravenous and oral pain medications.

4. Hernia: Patients are advised to avoid any strenuous activity for four to six weeks after surgery in an attempt to decrease the risk of this problem.

5. Intestinal obstruction (2 percent): Scar tissue can develop with healing after surgery, and this can result in intestinal blockage. Patients may present with abdominal bloating, pain, nausea, or vomiting. Conservative management may help to resolve this problem, but surgery to remove the scar tissue is occasionally necessary.

6. Prolonged ileus: This problem is a delay in the return of intestinal function which usually resolves spontaneously.

7. Ureteral injury: A rare occurrence which is usually managed at the time of surgery.

8. Accumulation of lymphatic fluid: Since lymph nodes and lymphatic tissue are removed during RPLND, lymph fluid can leak out of lymphatic vessels and form collections that may become symptomatic. These problems may require a change in the patient's diet or surgical drainage.

9. Pulmonary embolus (PE): During this operation, clots may form in the large veins around the kidneys. Rarely, these clots can break free and travel through the bloodstream to lodge in the lung, a condition known as a pulmonary embolus, which can be fatal.

10. Pneumonia: The risk of lung problems after RPLND is higher in patients who have been treated with chemotherapy first. Patients who undergo this procedure are instructed and encouraged to perform specific deep breathing exercises to try to avoid pneumonia or other lung problems post-operatively.

11. Damage to adjacent structures: Some other structures that may be inadvertently injured during this operation include blood vessels, intestines, liver, and spleen.

12. Infertility: The nerves that control emission and ejaculation (see Chapter 4) can be damaged during RPLND. As a result, until techniques to spare these nerves were developed, approximately 90 percent of patients who underwent RPLND were rendered infertile due to either failure of emission or retrograde ejaculation (see Chapter 7). These

patients were not impotent, just infertile, which was still an important problem since patients who develop testicular cancer tend to be in their reproductive years. In patients who are able to undergo the nerve-sparing RPLND, preservation of emission and ejaculation has been reported in up to 85 to 97 percent of cases. Unfortunately, palpable tumor in the lymph nodes is a contraindication to the nerve-sparing approach, so not everyone who undergoes a RPLND will be able to have the nerve-sparing procedure attempted.

13. Residual or recurrent tumor: Since the accuracy of current staging modalities is only 70 to 80 percent, some patients who undergo RPLND are found to have more disease than initially expected. In addition, follow-up studies may suggest recurrence of testicular cancer, by either rising tumor markers or abnormalities seen on chest x-ray, which will require additional treatment.

14. Death (less than 1 percent).

RPLND is a viable option for patients with low-stage nonseminomatous testicular cancer (i.e., Stage A, B1, or B2), as well as for patients with high-stage seminoma or NST, initially treated with chemotherapy, that are found to have a residual mass greater than 3 cm on follow-up CT scan.

Radiation Therapy

In this form of treatment, x-rays are focused on the lymph nodes in the groin and those in the abdominal area at the level of the kidneys to try to destroy residual cancer cells. Each treatment takes about 15 to 30 minutes, and the total dose of radiation is usually administered over a three-week period. After completing their course of therapy, patients are followed regularly by their urologist with blood work (i.e., AFP and B-HCG), chest x-ray, and CT scan of the abdomen.

Radiation therapy for testicular cancer is usually well tolerated with only mild short-term side effects (e.g., nausea or diarrhea) and a very low risk of long-term complications.

Seminomas are extremely sensitive to radiation, and therefore, radiation is a viable treatment option for low-stage seminoma (i.e., Stage A, B1, and B2). It is not adequate treatment for high-stage seminoma, and is not a good option for the treatment of nonseminomatous testicular tumors (NST).

Chemotherapy

Primarily because of effective chemotherapy, testicular cancer has become one of the most curable of all malignancies. Currently, the most successful chemotherapeutic protocols involve the intravenous administration of multiple drugs for a certain period of time. After each of the drugs is administered once, the patient is allowed time for the drugs to destroy cancer cells and for his body to recuperate from the side effects of the chemotherapy, and then, another round, or cycle, of drugs is administered. Three or four cycles of chemotherapy are usually given.

Side effects of chemotherapy include:

1. Decreased white blood cell counts, known as myelosuppression, which can impair a patient's ability to fight bacteria, thus resulting in life-threatening infections. Therefore, patient's blood counts are monitored closely while they are receiving chemotherapy.

2. Gastrointestinal problems, such as diarrhea or ulcers in the mouth.

3. Liver damage.

4. Infertility.

5. Residual or recurrent tumor.

6. Therapy-related leukemia (0.5 to 4 percent): There is a slight increased risk of developing leukemia some years after receiving chemotherapy for the treatment of testicular cancer.

7. Death: This is usually secondary to overwhelming infection.

Chemotherapy is a viable option for the treatment of patients with either high-stage seminoma or NST (i.e., stage B3 or C), or evidence of relapse of disease after RPLND or radiation therapy.

Some authors have suggested treating patients with B1 or B2 NST with chemotherapy instead of RPLND, and this remains a controversial issue.

Surveillance

This option involves no additional treatment after radical orchiectomy except for periodic reassessment with tumor markers (e.g., AFP and B-HCG), chest x-ray, and CT scan every one to three months for a few years, then every six months for a few years more, and once-a-year for a few years thereafter. Surveillance has been proposed for stage A seminomas and NST because of the complications associated with RPLND and the high salvage rates with chemotherapy.

This option requires reliable patients committed to the intense follow-up regimens. Surveillance is not an option for stage B or C disease.

TREATMENT BY CELL-TYPE AND STAGE

By this time, patients have already undergone radical orchiectomy and further staging studies. The information in this section is designed to serve as a guide for the various treatment options generally offered for the treatment of testicular cancer based on the cell-type and stage of the patient's disease. It is in no way meant to be taken as "urologic law."

Seminoma

At diagnosis, approximately 75 percent of patients will have disease confined to the testicle, 15 percent have lymph node involvement, and 10 percent will have distant metastasis.

Stage A

Adjuvant radiation therapy to the lymph nodes in the groin and around the kidney is usually recommended. Another option would be surveillance therapy, since only 8 to 10 percent of patients with clinical stage A can be expected to have undetected lymph node involvement. However, the rigid follow-up schedule required for surveillance therapy and the relative lack of morbidity associated with radiation therapy make this a controversial issue. Five-year survival rates (usually considered cure rates) for patients with stage A seminoma are approximately 93 to 100 percent.

Stage B1

Adjuvant radiation therapy is also recommended for this stage of seminoma with five-year survivals of 85 percent.

Stage B2

Adjuvant radiation therapy is also indicated in this stage with five-year survival rates also approximating 85 percent.

Stage B3

The use of radiation therapy alone in this stage results in five-year survivals of 65 percent, which are unacceptable. Therefore, the optimal treatment for these patients involves chemotherapy, with RPLND reserved for residual masses of greater than 3 cm on CT scan performed after the completion of chemotherapy. Using this approach, five-year survival rates are approximately 88 to 92 percent.

Stage C

Radiation therapy is not adequate treatment for this stage of disease. Primary chemotherapy, with RPLND reserved for patients with residual abdominal masses greater than 3 cm after chemotherapy, results in five-year survival rates approaching 88 to 92 percent.

Nonseminomas

At diagnosis, approximately 50 to 75 percent of patients will have disease outside the testicle, in either the lymph nodes or distant metastatic sites.

Stage A

A nerve-sparing RPLND is usually recommended for staging and therapeutic purposes. If tumor is found in the lymph nodes, it may be necessary to perform a more extensive lymph node dissection without sparing the nerves, and additional chemotherapy may be suggested. If, however, no residual cancer is found, observation with regular follow-up, as described prior, is usually all that is necessary. Five-year survival rates reported with this approach are approximately 100 percent. Patients who have recurrent disease after RPLND are treated with chemotherapy with cure rates also approaching 100 percent.

In light of the high success rate of chemotherapy for the treatment of testicular cancer, some authors have proposed surveillance therapy for patients with stage A NST. Opponents to surveillance therapy point out that clinical staging has a false-negative rate of 30 to 40 percent (i.e., patients may not manifest lymph node involvement on staging studies despite the presence of advanced disease), so approximately 30 to 40 percent of patients managed with surveillance therapy can be expected to develop recurrent disease, and 7 to 10 percent of these patients will succumb to their cancer. Surveillance therapy is contraindicated in those patients who are not reliable enough to keep all of their follow-up appointments.

Stage B1

A RPLND is usually recommended in this stage. If disease is microscopic, a nerve-sparing procedure is usually performed. If, however, obvious tumor is found at surgery, a more extensive lymph node dissection is performed without sparing the nerves. In addition, some physicians may recommend adjuvant chemotherapy after RPLND, while others may suggest close follow-up and reserve chemotherapy for those patients who develop recurrent disease (i.e., an option called observation with delayed chemotherapy). Five-year survivals in this stage approach 98 percent.

Stage B2

One option in this stage is a RPLND (not nerve-sparing due to the amount of disease) followed by either adjuvant chemotherapy or observation with delayed chemotherapy for those who relapse. Another option in this stage would be primary chemotherapy, reserving RPLND for those patients who fail to respond completely, as evidenced by either persistently elevated tumor markers or an abdominal mass greater than 3 cm on follow-up CT scan after chemotherapy. Five-year survival rates in this stage also approach 98 percent.

Stage B3

RPLND may be offered as the primary treatment with the subsequent use of adjuvant chemotherapy; however, given the amount of tumor in the lymph nodes in this stage, primary chemotherapy is usually recommended, with post-chemotherapy RPLND reserved for patients with bulky residual abdominal masses (i.e., greater than 3 cm). Five-year survival rates approach 80 percent in this stage.

Stage C

Primary chemotherapy is usually recommended. RPLND is reserved for patients with evidence of residual disease after chemotherapy. Five-year survival rates also approach 80 percent in this stage.

FERTILITY

Before the development of successful treatment options, survival was the most important concern when treating patients with testicular cancer, but now that the overall cure rate for this cancer approaches 97 percent, quality of life issues have become important. Fertility is one of these issues that needs to be addressed, since most of the patients who develop testicular cancer are in their reproductive years. Based on post-orchiectomy semen analyses, approximately 40 to 70 percent of patients have been found to be temporarily subfertile, and 25 percent of patients with testicular cancer will have a permanent, irreversible impairment of testicular reproductive function before any additional treatment for their cancer.

Radiation therapy does not appear to significantly affect long-term testicular function since 40 to 70 percent of patients who attempt to father children after radiation therapy for testicular cancer are able to achieve their goal. Of note, it may take up to one to two years after therapy for reproductive function to recover completely.

Approximately 76 percent of patients who attempt to father children after the nerve-sparing RPLND can be expected to have success. As a result, the surgical management of testicular cancer does not appear to significantly affect fertility unless the nerve-sparing procedure is not performed.

Unfortunately, chemotherapy significantly affects reproductive function. Only 30 percent of patients who attempt to father children after being treated with chemotherapy are successful.

Although the chances of achieving a successful pregnancy have improved with the nerve-sparing RPLND, patients with testicular cancer who desire to father children may still want to consider pre-operative or pre-treatment sperm banking, in case they require artificial insemination, or other reproductive techniques, to achieve this goal after definitive treatment of their disease.

Testicular cancer is curable, but you can't cure a problem unless you diagnose it first. One of the keys to the early diagnosis of testicular cancer is frequent self-examination of the genitalia. It is therefore recommended that men 15 to 45 years of age perform testicular self-examinations every one to two months, and if any suspicious lesions or changes are found, they should see a physician as soon as possible for further evaluation.

References

1. Foster RS and Donohue JP: "Fertility in Testicular Cancer Patients." *AUA Update Series* 1995; vol. 14, lesson 19.
2. Foster RS and Donohue JP: "Nerve-Sparing RPLND." *AUA Update Series* 1993; vol. 12, lesson 15.
3. Gardner E, Gray DJ, and O'Rahilly R: *Anatomy*, 4th ed. Philadelphia: WB Saunders Co., 1975.
4. Gillenwater JY, Grayhack JT, Howards SS, Duckett JW (eds.): *Adult and Pediatric Urology*, 3rd ed. St. Louis: Mosby, 1996.
5. Macfarlane MT: *Urology for the House Officer*, 2nd ed. Baltimore: Williams and Wilkins, 1995.
6. Richie JP: "Complications of Retroperitoneal Lymph Node Dissection." *AUA Update Series* 1993; vol. 12, lesson 16.
7. Roth BJ and Nichols CR: "Chemotherapy for Testicular Cancer: 1994." *AUA Update Series* 1994; vol. 13, lesson 22.
8. Wettlaufer JN: "The Management of Advanced Seminoma." *AUA Update Series* 1990; vol. 9, lesson 11.

CHAPTER 25

PENILE CANCER

As seen in Figure 25-1, the penis is made up of two corpora cavernosa, which are the shafts that fill with blood during the sexual act to give rise to an erection, and the corpus spongiosum, through which passes the urethra. These three structures are contained within a fibrous tissue called Buck's fascia. Superficial to this fascial layer lies the subcutaneous tissue which is covered by the skin of the penis.

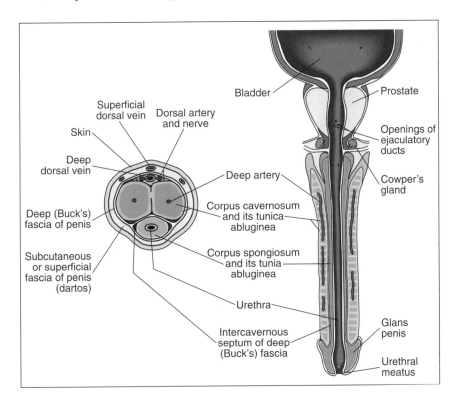

Figure 25-1: *Anatomy of the male reproductive system and cross-sectional view of the penis.*

A man's chances of developing cancer of the penis are similar to his chances of winning the lottery: one-in-a-million. In the United States, penile cancer is seen in 0.1 to 0.6 out of every 100,000 persons, accounting for one to six cases per million males. Since 99 percent of all penile cancers arise from the squamous cells that make up the skin of the penis, this chapter will deal specifically with squamous cell carcinoma of the penis (SCC).

Some of the factors that are believed to increase a person's risk of developing penile cancer include:

1. The presence of a foreskin: Penile cancer is extremely rare among populations that circumcise males in infancy; however, in countries where circumcision is not performed routinely, penile cancer is much more common. Therefore, circumcision at birth appears to protect against this type of cancer. On the other hand, inadequate or incomplete circumcision, where much of the foreskin remains, or circumcision performed after five years of age, is far less effective in preventing the development of penile cancer.

2. Phimosis: This is a condition in which the foreskin cannot be retracted to reveal the head of the penis (also known as the glans). Phimosis has been reported in 52 percent of patients diagnosed with penile cancer. It is believed that the inability to adequately cleanse the penis with a phimotic foreskin leads to chronic inflammation which may predispose to the development of SCC of the penis.

3. Poor hygiene: It has been suggested that inadequate cleansing of the uncircumcised penis creates optimal conditions for the action of, as yet, unknown agents that predispose patients to penile cancer.

4. Race: Penile cancer is more common in nonwhites than in whites.

5. Venereal disease: It has been suggested that the human papilloma virus (HPV) plays a significant role in the development of carcinoma of the penis (see Chapter 14).

6. Age: The risk of developing penile cancer appears to rise with increasing age, with most cases diagnosed in men between the ages of 60 to 69.

7. Cigarette smoking: The risk of penile cancer appears to be approximately three times greater in smokers than in nonsmokers.

8. Occupational exposure: It has been suggested that agricultural workers, painters, and men in jobs involving exposure to asbestos have an increased risk of developing cancer of the penis.

DIAGNOSIS

As with any disease process, the diagnosis of penile cancer involves the history obtained from the patient, a thorough physical examination, and certain laboratory tests and special studies.

History

Patients typically complain of a penile mass, lump, or nodule which may be ulcerated, and these lesions may bleed occasionally. The average age at diagnosis is 60 years. Patients may report having had multiple infections involving the foreskin and/or glans, a condition known as balanoposthitis.

Penile cancer is noteworthy for delays in patient presentation to the physician, possibly due to embarrassment about the location of the lesion. Therefore, the average time interval between the patient's initial perception of a penile lesion and his presentation to a physician is ten months.

Physical Examination

Examination of the genitalia in these patients usually reveals a lesion on the glans, or head of the penis, in 48 percent of cases, on the foreskin in 21 percent, involving both the glans and the foreskin in 9 percent, and in the groove behind the glans (i.e., the coronal sulcus) in 6 percent of the cases. The penile shaft is rarely the site of origin of a penile cancer, but it can be involved by direct extension of tumors that originate on the glans or foreskin. Although retraction of a phimotic foreskin may not be possible, occasionally a nodular lesion may be palpable beneath the foreskin.

The first sites to which penile cancer spreads when it progresses beyond the penis are the lymph nodes in the inguinal (i.e., groin) area; therefore, the physician will examine the inguinal lymph nodes for evidence of enlargement. Approximately 50 percent of patients with penile cancer will be found to have enlarged inguinal lymph nodes, but in only half of these is the enlargement due to the spread of cancer, while in the other half, the enlargement is due to inflammation. It should also be noted that approximately 20 percent of patients with penile cancer involving their inguinal lymph nodes have no palpable enlargement of those nodes.

Laboratory Studies

Presently, there is no blood test available that can diagnose penile cancer. Blood tests can be used to evaluate the function of the liver (i.e., liver function tests or LFTs) in an attempt to search for evidence of metastatic spread of cancer to a patient's liver, and therefore, LFTs may be performed in the evaluation of patients with penile cancer.

Penile Biopsy

Many conditions can cause a penile lesion, and since there are no physical characteristics that will allow an unequivocal diagnosis, the definitive diagnosis of penile cancer requires a biopsy of the lesion. This can be performed in the office under local anesthesia. A piece of the penile lesion is removed and sent to the pathologist for microscopic evaluation. It may require a small dissolvable suture to close the biopsy site.

It usually takes about four to seven days for the biopsy results to return, and the possibilities include:

- *No evidence of cancer.* This is great news. There are a variety of benign conditions that can result in suspicious penile lesions requiring a biopsy. Some of these conditions may require further treatment, while others may not.

- *The biopsy shows cancer.* At this point in time, the patient will follow-up with his urologist to discuss the options available for the treatment of his penile cancer. Three areas are usually addressed : 1) treatment of the penile lesion, 2) management of inguinal lymph nodes, and 3) treatment of metastatic disease (i.e., cancer that has spread to organs far beyond the penis), if present.

TREATMENT OF THE PRIMARY CANCER

This means treatment of the cancerous lesion involving the penis itself. Adequate tumor control is crucial to prevent or halt the spread of the cancer beyond the penis. Although surgical removal of part, or all, of the penis can result in a variety of problems, ranging from the loss of body image and sexual function to the loss of the ability to urinate in the standing position, one thing is certain: cancer of the penis must be treated, since without treatment, only 6 percent of patients survive three years and only 3 percent of patients can be expected to survive five years.

Carcinoma in situ (CIS) is a form of cancer of the penis confined to the skin layer. Various treatment options exist for CIS of the penis including: 1) local excision, 2) fulgaration (or destruction) of the lesion with electrical devices or laser therapy, 3) radiation therapy, or 4) application of chemotherapeutic cream. Lesions that fail to respond to less invasive forms of treatment require local excision.

Except for CIS, the primary lesion of penile cancer is usually best treated by wide surgical excision leaving adequate tumor-free margins (i.e., the tumor is excised along with 2 cm of normal-appearing tissue). Lesions confined to the foreskin may be managed with circumcision alone (see Chapter 1). Patients with tumors confined to the glans or distal part of the penile shaft may be treated adequately with removal of only a portion of the penis (partial penectomy). However, when the cancer involves the proximal shaft or base of the penis (the part of the penis close to the patient's body), or when the extent of disease prevents the performance of a partial penectomy with adequate tumor-free margins (2 cm), then, the entire penis is usually removed (total penectomy) and the patient urinates via an opening made in the perineum, which is the area of the body located between the scrotum and the anus.

Penectomy, either partial or total, is the most common surgical treatment for the penile lesion of cancer of the penis. The patient is advised not to take any aspirin, ibuprofen, or other blood-thinners for at least one week before surgery in an attempt to decrease the risk of excessive bleeding during or after the procedure, and to abstain from eating and drinking after midnight on the night before surgery. He is admitted to the hospital on the day of the procedure which is usually performed under general or spinal anesthesia.

The lesion is covered with the finger of a surgical glove to try to prevent spillage of tumor cells as the penis is manipulated. The skin of the penis is incised circumferentially, and then, the corpora cavernosa and corpus spongiosum are transected in guillotine fashion approximately 2 cm proximal to the lesion in an attempt to assure adequate tumor-free margins. The opening of the urethra, known as the urethral meatus, is then remodeled, and a urinary catheter is placed for bladder drainage. This catheter is usually removed in one to three days.

In order for the patient to urinate in the standing position and have a functional penile stump, his penis needs to be at least 3 cm long after surgery. If residual penile length after surgery will be insufficient to allow the patient to direct his urinary stream, or if the cancer involves the proximal shaft or prevents the performance of a partial penectomy with an adequate margin, total penectomy is usually performed with removal of the entire penis and diversion of the urethra to the perineum. In this case, the patient will also have a temporary drain placed under the skin in the scrotal area to prevent fluid accumulation, in addition to the urinary catheter for bladder drainage. This skin drain is usually removed in three to five days, depending on the volume of drainage. The urinary catheter is usually left in place for approximately one week to allow ample time for healing. On rare occasions, the decision of whether to perform partial or total penectomy can only be made at the time of surgery, and patients are usually made aware of this possibility before surgery to treat their penile cancer.

Penectomy, either partial or total, usually requires 30 to 60 minutes with slightly more time needed to remove the entire penis. Patients are usually able to eat a regular diet as soon as they are alert, and are kept comfortable with pain medication. They are usually discharged home one to two days after the operation with oral antibiotics and pain medication, and can generally resume daily activities in about one to two weeks.

Complications after partial or total penectomy are rare, but include:

1. Infection: The risk of this problem has been reduced by the use of antibiotics for two to six weeks after surgery.
2. Bleeding.
3. Pain: Post-operative pain can usually be controlled with oral pain medication.

4. Urethral stricture: Scar tissue may cause narrowing at the urethral meatus, and this problem may require periodic dilation of this opening to prevent voiding problems.

5. Residual or recurrent tumor: Local recurrence of tumor in the penis is rare after partial or total penectomy (i.e., approximately ten percent); however, approximately one-third of patients, regardless of their physical examination, will have inguinal lymph node involvement which will require additional treatment.

6. Anesthetic risk, such as heart attack or death, which are rare in healthy patients.

After the surgery, the specimen is sent to the pathologist for microscopic examination. Before recommendations for further treatment can be made, the aggressiveness of the patient's cancer and whether or not it has spread outside the penis must be determined.

GRADE

The pathology report usually describes the grade, or degree of differentiation, of the cancer cells. Grading uses the microscopic appearance of the tumor cells to predict how aggressive, or fast-growing, they are. Tumors in which the cells closely resemble normal penile cells are described as well differentiated cancers and tend to be less aggressive, while tumors made up of cells that do not resemble normal penile cells are called poorly differentiated cancers and are assumed to be very aggressive. Tumor cells with features between these two extremes are described as moderately differentiated and tend to have intermediate aggressiveness. A numerical system is often used to grade cancers, with grade I tumors being well differentiated, grade II tumors being moderately differentiated, and grade III tumors being poorly differentiated.

Patient survival appears to be inversely related to the grade of the tumor; that is, the higher the grade, the lower the survival rate.

STAGE

Stage refers to the degree of invasion, or in other words, how deep the cancer has penetrated into the penis, or how far it has spread into the surrounding tissues or to other parts of the body, if at all. Accurate staging, combined with other data available at diagnosis, helps the urologist assess the patient's prognosis and make rational treatment recommendations.

There are two staging systems for penile cancer in common use: the original system described by Jackson and the more recent TNM classification, which stands for T - tumor, N - nodes (i.e., lymph node involvement), and M - metastasis (i.e., distant spread of cancer).

In the Jackson system:

- **Stage I** tumor is confined to the glans or foreskin.
- **Stage II** cancers extend onto the shaft of the penis, without obvious lymph node involvement.
- **Stage III** cancers have spread to the inguinal lymph nodes, and the amount of disease appears to be treatable with surgical removal of these nodes.
- **Stage IV** tumors either invade adjacent structures, such as the prostate or urethra, or have spread to distant sites (e.g., lung, liver, bone, or brain).

In the TNM classification:

- **T0** signifies that no cancer is found in the penis.
- **Tis** refers to carcinoma in situ.
- **T1** tumor invades the subcutaneous tissue.
- **T2** cancers invade the corpora cavernosa or the corpus spongiosum.
- **T3** tumors have extended into the prostate or the urethra.
- **T4** cancers invade other structures in the area of the penis.
- **N0** means that no cancer is found in the lymph nodes.
- **N1** signifies that penile cancer has spread to one inguinal lymph node.
- **N2** signifies the presence of cancer spread in multiple inguinal lymph nodes on either side or both sides of the patient.
- **N3** disease involves lymph nodes deep within the inguinal area or in the pelvis (i.e., the pelvic lymph nodes).
- **M0** indicates the absence of distant spread of disease.

- **M1** signifies that the cancer has spread to distant sites (e.g., lung, liver, bone, or brain).

As stated earlier, pathologic examination of the specimen removed in the treatment of the penile lesion will help to stage the cancer. There are other "non-invasive" methods that may also be used to clinically stage the patient's disease in an attempt to help guide treatment recommendations.

Physical Examination of the Inguinal Lymph Nodes

Palpable inguinal lymph nodes suggest the presence of cancer spread; however, although 50 percent of patients with penile cancer will be found to have palpable inguinal lymph nodes at the time of diagnosis, only 1/2 of these patients will truly have spread of disease to their inguinal nodes. In the other half of these patients, the lymph node enlargement is due to an inflammatory reaction rather than cancerous involvement. Therefore, patients are usually treated with antibiotics for two to six weeks after partial or total penectomy, and then, the urologist re-evaluates the inguinal lymph nodes. Lymph nodes that are palpable after a course of antibiotics are highly suggestive of lymphatic involvement with penile cancer which requires further treatment. The problem is that approximately 20 percent of patients with penile cancer will have lymph node involvement without palpable enlargement.

Liver Function Tests (LFTs)

Liver function tests (LFTs) are blood tests used to search for abnormalities in the liver which could suggest the presence of metastatic disease involving the liver.

Chest X-ray

The chest x-ray (CXR) study is used to screen for the presence of metastatic disease involving the lungs.

Computed Axial Tomography Scan (CT scan)

This is an x-ray study in which the patient lies on a table that is passed through a circular machine that, with the help of a computer, makes cross-sectional images of the body. It is used to search for enlarged lymph nodes or for evidence of metastatic disease. Since an iodine-based contrast solution is administered intravenously to help visualize certain structures, the risks of CT scan are similar to those of IVP (see Chapter 18).

Magnetic Resonance Imaging Scan (MRI)

This study uses magnetic waves, instead of x-rays, to take pictures of the patient's internal organs. The patient is usually required to lie still in a tube-shaped chamber for 30 to 40 minutes which can be a difficult task for claustrophobic patients. Magnetic resonance imaging (MRI) can be used in place of CT scan.

Once the grade and clinical stage of the patient's cancer have been estimated, the urologist usually presents the information to the patient and discusses the options available to further manage the patient's disease. Points that are usually addressed include: 1) treatment of the inguinal lymph nodes, and 2) treatment of metastatic disease, if present.

TREATMENT OF INGUINAL LYMPH NODES

As stated earlier, the first site to which penile cancer spreads beyond the penis is usually the inguinal lymph nodes. Metastatic spread of tumor cells through the bloodstream to distant sites may occur, but this rarely occurs early in the course of the disease. Lymph nodes that are palpable after a two to six week course of antibiotics are presumed to be involved with cancer, and require further treatment. Patients without palpable lymph nodes may still have undetected spread of penile cancer.

The stage of the primary tumor gives some insight into the chances of lymph node involvement. For example, patients with stage Tis or T1 disease have a 5 percent chance of lymph node spread, whereas those with tumor stage T2 or higher have a 60 percent chance of lymph node involvement.

The grade of a patient's cancer also helps the urologist estimate the risk of lymph node spread from penile cancer. Patients with poorly differentiated tumors have a greater risk of having their lymph nodes involved with spread from penile cancer than those with well differentiated tumors.

Two options exist for the management of the inguinal lymph nodes.

Observation

This option involves regular follow-up visits to the urologist with physical examination of the inguinal area, CXR, and CT scan every one to two months for two years, then every six months for two years, and then once-a-year for a few more years. In the time between physician visits, the patient is instructed to perform self-examinations of the inguinal areas as well. The development of palpable lymph nodes is suggestive of recurrent disease and requires definitive treatment to remove the lymph nodes involved with cancer.

Observation is an option for patients with well differentiated penile cancers less than stage T2 and without palpable lymph nodes.

Inguinal Lymph Node Dissection

Inguinal lymph node dissection (ILND) involves the surgical removal of lymphatic tissue in the inguinal, or groin, area in an attempt to excise residual penile cancer which has spread to the inguinal lymph nodes and thus, cure the patient's disease.

In an attempt to optimize conditions for the procedure, certain preparatory steps are usually taken:

- Patients are usually treated with a two to six week course of antibiotics after removal of the penile tumor in an attempt to decrease the risk of wound infection.

- Since removal of lymphatic tissue may predispose patients to leg swelling by delaying the lymphatic drainage from the lower extremities, patients may be measured for waist-high stockings which will be worn post-operatively to try to decrease this leg swelling.

The patient is admitted on the morning of surgery. The procedure is usually performed under general or spinal anesthesia. Incisions are made in the inguinal area just below the crease where the thigh meets the trunk. Then, all of the fat and lymphatic tissue between the skin and the muscles of the thigh is removed from the inguinal area and upper thigh. Multiple operations have been designed to remove different amounts of lymphatic tissue depending on the grade and stage of the patient's disease in an attempt to achieve a curative effect while minimizing morbidity. After the lymphatic tissue has been removed, suction catheters are placed in this area to prevent fluid accumulation under the remaining flaps of skin, and the incision is closed.

The decision to perform ILND on the side of the penile lesion or bilaterally depends on various factors, including the presence of palpable disease and the stage of the patient's cancer. However, since up to 60 percent of patients with lymph node involvement in one groin will have cancer involving the other side as well, if cancer is found in one inguinal area at the time of ILND, it is recommended that the contralateral groin also undergo ILND. Removal of lymph nodes from deep within the pelvis (i.e., pelvic lymph node dissection) is recommended for young, healthy individuals with tumor involving the inguinal lymph nodes.

ILND usually takes 60 to 90 minutes per side. After the procedure, patients are kept at bedrest for approximately one week to allow the incisions to begin healing before patients resume ambulation. Suction catheters are kept in place until all skin drainage ceases (usually one week). Patients are instructed to wear their waist-high compression stockings for at least six months. Post-operatively, antibiotics are used in an attempt to prevent wound infection, and patients are kept comfortable with oral pain medication. The usual hospital stay is seven to ten days. Patients can usually resume normal activities in a few weeks.

ILND is a procedure with a high morbidity. It has an overall complication rate of 50 percent. Some of the possible side effects from the operation include:

1. Infection (10 percent).
2. Bleeding.
3. Pain.
4. Lymphedema (10 to 16 percent): This is persistent swelling of the lower extremities due to decreased lymphatic drainage.
5. Lymphocele (10 percent): This is a subcutaneous collection of lymph fluid that may occasionally need to be drained.
6. Prolonged drain output: Occasionally, the drains placed under the skin to prevent fluid collections continue to put out lymph fluid or blood for

longer periods than usual. This usually resolves with conservative management.

7. Deep vein thrombosis and/or pulmonary embolus (5 percent): During ILND, patients lie on the operating table for one to two hours while the urologist performs surgery around blood vessels in the legs. As a result, clots can form in the veins that drain the legs, a condition known as deep vein thrombosis (DVT). Symptoms of DVT can include asymmetric swelling or pain in the legs, but DVT can be present without symptoms. Sometimes, these clots can break free and travel through the bloodstream to lodge in the lungs, a potentially fatal condition known as a pulmonary embolus (PE). Blood-thinners are sometimes used in the period around this operation to try to decrease the risk of these complications.

8. Damage to adjacent structures, such as blood vessels and nerves.

9. Residual or recurrent disease.

10. Necrosis of the flaps of skin in the area of dissection (20 to 30 percent): This is a significant complication which may require skin grafting to repair the resulting defect.

11. Death (3 percent).

ILND is a therapeutic procedure resulting in five-year disease-free survival rates of 50 to 60 percent in patients with lymph node involvement as compared to almost certain death if untreated. Some authors have reported that additional chemotherapy after an ILND revealing multiple lymph nodes involved with tumor, may improve five-year disease-free survivals up to 82 percent. ILND is indicated in patients with penile cancer who have either:

• Persistently palpable inguinal lymph nodes after a two to six week course of antibiotics following treatment of their penile lesion

• Tumor stage T2 or higher, regardless of grade; or

• Moderately or poorly differentiated tumor, despite a low tumor stage.

Patients with a significant amount of tumor involving the deep pelvic nodes, or with tumor spread involving the lymph nodes in the abdominal area, have a poor prognosis. Since ILND is not believed to alter survival in patients with this degree of disease, it is usually not recommended in these patients.

In summary, although the patient tends to be most concerned about the treatment of his penile lesion, the status and management of the lymph nodes in the inguinal area is the most important determinant of the patient's survival. After treatment of the penile lesion and further staging, there is general agreement that patients with Tis, grade I lesions and no palpable lymph nodes may be managed with observation therapy. It also seems to be agreed upon that patients with penile cancers of any T stage and resectable inguinal lymph nodes which remain palpable following a course of antibiotic therapy should undergo some form of ILND. Large fixed lymph node disease is believed to be associated with incurable disease not amenable to surgical therapy. The dilemma for nodal treatment involves patients with invasive penile cancers (i.e., T1 or higher) with impalpable lymph nodes. As stated prior, patients with moderately or poorly differentiated tumors are usually advised to undergo ILND. Patients with well differentiated T1 disease are usually managed with observation therapy; however, an ILND is also an option in this case. Due to the increased risk of lymph node involvement in the higher T stages, patients with stage T2, T3, or T4 disease are usually advised to undergo ILND regardless of the grade of their cancer.

Radiation therapy has been tried in patients with lymph node spread of their disease, but it is measurably less effective than ILND.

TREATMENT OF METASTATIC DISEASE

In patients whose penile cancer has spread to distant sites, such as the lungs, liver, bone, or brain, chemotherapy using multiple drugs appears to offer the best hope for survival. However, responses have generally been short-lived. In addition, the side effects of these chemotherapeutic agents are significant, and include 1) decreased white blood cell count which can impair a person's ability to fight infection; 2) gastrointestinal problems, such as diarrhea; 3) liver damage; and 4) death, usually secondary to overwhelming infections.

PROGNOSIS

Penile cancer appears to be a surgical disease since the best chance for cure seems to involve excision of the penile lesion, followed by the surgical removal of local lymph nodes, if indicated. Once disease spreads beyond the inguinal lymph nodes, the chances for cure are significantly decreased. Table 25-1 demonstrates the five-year survival rates of patients definitively treated for penile cancer based on the stage of disease at diagnosis.

Table 25-1: Survival Rates for Penile Cancer Based on the Stage of Disease at Diagnosis	
Stage	5-Year Survival (% of Patients)
I	90-97
II	60-90
III	50-60
IV	0-20

Penile cancer is curable if it is diagnosed early in the course of the disease. The smaller the lesion, the easier it will be to treat with a lower chance of significant residual penile deformity. Therefore, any patient with a penile lesion should see a physician for further evaluation.

References

1. Gillenwater JY, Grayhack JT, Howards SS, and Duckett JW (eds.): *Adult and Pediatric Urology*, 3rd ed. St. Louis: Mosby, 1996.
2. Lynch DF and Schellhammer PF: "Contemporary Concepts in Ilioinguinal Lymphadenectomy for Squamous Cell Carcinoma of the Penis." *AUA Update Series* 1997; vol. 16, lesson 33.
3. Macfarlane MT: *Urology for the House Officer*, 2nd ed. Baltimore: Williams and Wilkins, 1995.
4. Mukamel E and deKernion JB: "Early Versus Delayed Lymph Node Dissection Versus No Lymph Node Dissection for Carcinoma of the Penis." *AUA Update Series* 1990; vol. 9, lesson 2.
5. Thompson IM and Fair WR: "Penile Carcinoma." *AUA Update Series* 1990; vol. 9, lesson 1.

EPILOGUE

An epilogue is defined as a closing section added to a novel, play, etc., providing further comment. The final "bottom line" of this book is taken from *The ABC's of Prostate Cancer* by Oesterling and Moyad: "An objective and knowledgeable patient combined with an objective and knowledgeable doctor creates the strongest and most beneficial force in medicine."

Nothing is perfect. Time constraints in the office prevent physicians from spending as much time as they'd like answering their patients' questions. In addition, given the complicated nature of some of these topics, it is impossible to teach everything there is to know about them in a short book. Although this book is not meant to substitute for the services of a physician, my hope is that it will give people who read it more insight into certain urologic disease processes, and this insight may allow them to seek medical attention sooner—or at least will help them to deal better with treatment decisions that need to be made.

Dealing with everyday life and aging is difficult enough, but the added stress of having to deal with a health problem can sometimes make life seem unbearable. Almost every issue addressed in this book can be frightening. Added to this is the social "taboo" associated with discussing issues relating to reproduction and the genitalia, which can make anybody feel that they have no one to turn to for information about these "sensitive" topics.

The last chapters of this book, which discussed the clinical aspects of some of the more common urologic cancers, fail to really address the emotional aspects associated with dealing with these diseases that patients and their families must try to cope with everyday; however, this does not mean that these emotional aspects are any less important.

Hopefully, if a person with a urologic problem reads this book, he'll realize that he's not alone.There are many places set up to help men with urologic problems, and many places to support their loved ones as well. People can usually start by seeking information at their local hospital or nearby university centers. In addition, following this section, I have included a brief list of support groups and organizations, as well as some internet addresses, that readers may use to try to obtain more information.

I hope that the information that I've collected here goes a long way in helping the reader achieve urologic good health.

RESOURCES

The following list of organizations includes street addresses, telephone numbers and internet addresses, where available.

American Cancer Society (ACS)

(800) ACS-2345
www.cancer.org
(Select "Cancer Information" to find basic material on many types of cancer, including penile, testicular, bladder and prostate.)

American Foundation for Urologic Disease (AFUD)

1128 North Charles Street
Baltimore, MD 21201-5506
(410) 468-1800
www.afud.org

American Urological Association (AUA)

1120 North Charles Street
Baltimore, MD 21201-5559
(410) 727-1100
www.auanet.org

Health Information Network, Inc.

231 Market Place, No. 331
San Ramon, CA 94583
(925) 358-4370

Mednets

www.internets.com/urology.htm
(Can be used to obtain clinical information regarding various urologic problems as well as suggestions for other web sites that may be of help)

National Cancer Institute (NCI)
Public Inquiries Office
Building 31, Room 10A16
Bethesda, MD 20892-2580
(800) 4-CANCER
www.nci.nih.gov

National Institute on Aging Information Center
P.O. Box 8057
Gaithersburg, MD 20898-8057
(800) 222-2225
www.nih.gov/nia/
(click on health information)

National Kidney and Urologic Diseases Information Clearinghouse
3 Information Way
Bethesda, MD 20892-3580
(301) 651-4415
www.niddk.nih.gov/health/kidney/nkudic.htm

National Register of Health Service Providers in Psychology
1120 G Street NW, Suite 330
Washington, DC 20005
(202) 783-7663
www.nationalregister.com

Nidus Information Services
175 Fifth Avenue, Suite 2338
New York, NY 10010
(800) 334-9355
www.well-connected.com

Patient Advocates for Advanced Cancer Treatments (PAACT)

1143 Parmelee NW
Grand Rapids, MI 49504
(616) 453-1477
www.osz.com/paact/
(provides information about prostate cancer exclusively)

Sexual Information and Education Council of the United States

130 West 42nd Street
New York, NY 10036-7802
(212) 819-9770
www.siecus.org

INDEX

U

ABOUT THE AUTHOR

Angelo S. Paola, M.D., graduated from State University of New York–Stony Brook Medical School in 1986 and received his urologic training at West Virginia University. He is a board certified urologist, and with his partners Robert L. Karp, M.D. and James E. Alver, M.D., Dr. Paola treats patients at Bay Area Urological Associates in Brandon, Florida. He is a member of the American Urological Association and a fellow of the American College of Surgeons. Dr. Paola has numerous publications in the field of urology. In addition to the practice of urology, he has devoted himself to educating physicians and the general public in various aspects of urology.